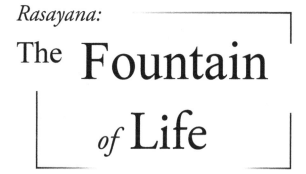

*Rasayana:*

The Fountain

*of* Life

_Rasayana:_

The Fountain

_of_ Life

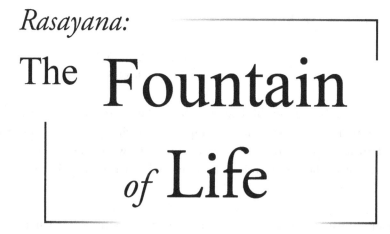

Dr. Mayank S. Vora

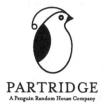

PARTRIDGE

A Penguin Random House Company

Print information available on the last page.

**To order additional copies of this book, contact**
Partridge India
000 800 10062 62
orders.india@partridgepublishing.com

www.partridgepublishing.com/india

# CONTENTS

**Part 3 Classical Rasayana**

**Part 4 Medium of Transport**

To

My Father Late Sudhirkant Maneklal Vora

# PREFACE

Human body is one of the most exciting nature's miracles. It is very complex multicellular organism in which the survival and health depends upon proper organization, coordination and harmony between self and surroundings. After birth, growth and senility ultimately leading to death are inevitable processes. It is correctly stated that aging begins before birth and continues throughout life at different rates, in different races for different individuals and for different tissues of the body. Aging represent structural and functional changes of an organism over its entire life span.

Health is an important factor in attaining individual goal, whether it is wealth or happiness, material or spiritual or indeed moksha. The modern age is characterized by pressures, hurry, worry, the pressures of making a quick buck and temptations of corruption. These are bound to deviations from the safe routines of diet and habit.

In India the science of *Ayurveda* is probably the first on this planet to describe the science of life, its central theme being efforts to protect life from disease and aging. *Ayurveda* is natural and universal therapy since the time immemorial, fulfilling the aims and goals with positive health of human being. It is still in practice worldwide in different different forms and acceptance of Ayurvedic regimen and phyto-therapy are increasing day- by-day. Rasayana is one of the eight clinical specialties of classical *Ayurveda*.

Rasayana is not a drug therapy but is a specialized procedure practiced in the form of rejuvenative recipes, dietary regimen and special health promoting conduct and behavior i.e., Achara-Rasayana. Rasayana means the way for attaining excellent rasa i.e. one attains longevity, memory, intelligence, freedom from disorder, youthful age, excellence of luster, complexion and voice, optimum strength of physique and sense organs, alleviates diseases, successful words, respectability and brilliance. Everybody desires and has right to remain healthy and avoid sickness to enjoy life, to achieve the desired goal and dreams.

Health is maintained by improving immunity of the body against diseases. This could be achieved by administering Rasayana herbs. Rasayana therapy was practiced as an independent clinical discipline as a positive health medicine. With passage of time this important branch of knowledge has ceased to be in practice in its appropriate form.

Panchakarma therapy primarily aims at cleansing the body of its accumulated impurities and nourishing the tissues. Once this achieved, it becomes very easy to rejuvenate these tissues by administering appropriate Rasayana herb and prevent the process of aging. The span of life thus prolonged and the individual leads a disease free old age. He/she becomes capable of serving the society with his accumulated experience without any mental disability and physical delay.

There are numbers of excellent books on Rasayana therapy available but a book written from common man perspective is missing. Hence attempt is made to write simple book, which everyone can easily read and put it in practice.

This book is divided in four parts. First part deals with introduction of *Ayurveda*, antioxidation therapy, free radicals and their source, supplements and their role in disease prevention; Rasayana therapy, diet and Lifestyle, and herbs and their influence on our health. Second part provides detailed account of different single herb Rasayana, which includes Amalaki, *Aloe vera*, Ashoka, Ashwagandha, Bala, Bibhitaki, Bhallataka, Brahmi, Guduchi, Ginger, Gotu kola, Guggulu, Rasona, Shatavari, Haritaki, Shankhpushpi, Vedanta, Punarnava, Haridra, Nagkeshar, Musta, Twak and Yashtimadhu. The third part covers most important and popular classical Rasayana i.e. Brahma Rasayana, Chyawanprash and Triphala. The last part includes Ghee and Honey, the medium of transport of Rasayana.

The book will give an idea about Ayurvedic concepts and aspect of preventive and curative treatments. This book is specifically written for the ordinary common man and provides useful information about Rasayana therapy and its role in maintaining sound health and longevity.

The book does not require reader to possess any prior knowledge of Rasayana. It aims at providing reader sufficient knowledge to use the information and techniques of Rasayana to improve his or her life and consciousness on all levels. A glossary of terms has been included for ease in using this book.

The knowledge supplied in this book will be of lasting value to everyone including foreign visitors who come here for rejuvenation therapy. It will serve as ready reckoner for them. I hope that all readers of this book will find information not only very helpful but also a source of inspiration that will lead others to expand on the ideas presented herein. Readers who wish to know the *Ayurveda* and Rasayana therapy in further details can look at the recommended list for future reading. In the meantime, I hope you find this book useful, interesting and fascinating.

Please write to me about questions and comments at msvora2003@ gmail.com

Vadodara
Dr. Mayank S. Vora

# ACKNOWLEDGEMENTS

First and foremost, I express my gratitude to Parma Pujya Swami Viditatmanandji for his divine blessings has made this publication a reality.

I would like to thank my wife Dipti, not only for sharing the vision and providing the motivation to make this book become reality, but in addition for her continuing support for going through this book with care and indulgence.

How can I forget my sons Hirak and Nehal, not only they made arrangement for the publication, but provided moral support and encouragement at every stage during the preparation of manuscript. Thank you for understanding how important it has been for me to write this book. Thank you also to my daughter in laws Dipa and Tarjani and little Rishi and Ashni.

I thank whole my family and friends for providing me all kind of help and support during the course of this book.

Our Vedas, Charak Samhita, Sushruta Samhita have immense wisdom that can guide us for keeping good health and maintaining mental equilibrium. I am indebted to ancient sages as well as sages of our time who brought this wisdom for us.

I am grateful to the authors of number of books, journals without which there would be nothing to support my words.

I am obliged to Maveric Pana, Ann Minoza and Joe Anderson, Partridge India, a Penguin Randsom House Company for having printed this book in short time.

Finally, I would like to express my gratitude to my mother Smt Bakulben S. Vora for her love and affection.

I am really thankful to my friends, well-wishers for their sincere support by way of thoughts, words and deed.

# PART I

# INTRODUCTION

# CHAPTER 1

## *Ayurveda:* **An Ancient Universal Healing System**

"In reality it is not bacteria themselves that produce the disease, but we believe it is the chemical constituents of these microorganisms enacting upon unbalanced cell metabolism of the human body that actually produces the disease. We also believe that if the metabolism of human body is perfectly balanced or poised, it is susceptible to no disease."

Royal Rafe

*Ayurveda* which means science of life and longevity. It is the oldest medical science in the Indian subcontinent and has been practiced in India, Sri Lanka and Asian countries since 10ᵗʰ centuy BC. It has a sound philosophical and experiential basis. It is not easy to decide the exact period of origin of *Ayurveda*. Because it is not the contribution a single individual and of few years. But it is a contribution of thousands of sages through centuries. *Ayurveda* originated in heavan from Lord Brahma (creator of universe)then transferred to Ashwinikumars who transmitted to Lord Indra, at later date rishi Charak, Sushruta and Vagbhatta wrote Charak samhita (5ᵗʰ century BC), Sushruta Samhita(6ᵗʰ and 5ᵗʰ Century BC) and Ashtanga Hridaya (7ᵗʰ Century AD), respectively. Charaka, Susrutha and Vagbhatta are considered the pioneer ancient scholars who contributed much to the development of *Ayurveda* through their compilations, interpretations and experiments in *Ayurveda*. It was Charak who gave for the first time the medical history, the principles of immunity, metabolism, embriology etc. Charak's knowledge on anatomy and various organs of human body was astonishing. He gave the fundamentals of ayurvedic treatments and detailed description of herbs and their importance in health. Considering the tremendous contribution, Charak is considered "father of medicines"; while Sushruta developed around 125 types of surgical instruments including scalpels, needles mostly designed from the jaws of animals and used horse's hair as stiching thread. He developed protocols for 300 surgical operations. Considering his enormous contribution in the field of human surgery Sushrutra is known as "father of surgery". *Ayurveda* is evolved with a intension to have a happy human life, free from diseases long life. Rishis revealed the deepest truths related to human anatomy, physiology, psychology, health, diseases and their managements. Remember at that time no CT scan, MRI and sonography were available. *Ayurveda* is a complete science. It is a qualitative holistic science of health and longevity. It is universally fact that everybody wants to live long with sound health. No body wants to become old and die. Our desire for longevity is mentioned in "Atharvaveda". There is an in built desire of every individual to live for 100 years and more and that too in healthy state of body, mind and, all sense organs especially vision and hearing. A long healthy life has been the cherished desire of man since ancient times. In this stressful, over-busy and toxic world, our natural health, happiness and the inner sense of well-being are masked by the accumulation of impurities. These impurities or toxins called *ama* causes deterioration of normal body functioning. A rejuvenation therapy can revitalize senses, detoxify the body, restore good health and young look and even increase resistance to diseases. Ancient texts say that rejuvenation therapy can bring back the youthfulness long after one has past that age and it can also increase the life span by many years. Rejuvenation therapy is known to have cured chronic diseases for which otherwise it was impossible to find any treatment.

If you want to live a long healthy active life free from diseases, apart from following Ayurvedic lifestyle, you should also explore other ways of achieving this aim. Regular exercise is one of the most effective ways of overcoming a number of age related problems. To keep your body physically fit and moving the following exercises are recommended.

- ❖ Light gym exercises
- ❖ Surya Namaskar
- ❖ Yoga
- ❖ Dancing

- ❖ Swimming
- ❖ Aerobics
- ❖ Gentle weight lifting

Suitable nutrition should also be high on your priority. There is a growing tendency in modern times to make the diet as pleasing to the eyes as possible and tasty to the taste buds ingloring to their ultimate effect on health. This has lead to the refining of cereals and sugar and addition of salts to various food stuffs to make them tasty and delicious. Remember all antiaging treatments are a matter of balance between administration of appropriate Rasayana, balanced diet, regular exercises and stress free Lifestyle. Our organs are created to live over 300 years provided right nourishment is received and sufficient care is taken. Today in overbusy world no body has got time visit gym regularly or to think about food, so wear tear occur rapidly as a result signs of aging are noticed.

In addition to good nutrition, exercise, mental attitudes and positive thinking are also essential in fighting aging. There is no point in taking a few antioxidant pills and doing some exercise, when your brain remains neglected and your thoughts become vivid.

This is only possible when a person remain free from disease by taking adequate measures.

## Importance of Rasayana Therapy

Acharya Charak has categorically mentioned that with short span of our life and non-healthy state of living, one cannot achieve moksha which is the ultimate goal of life. Acharya Charak said that one should give utmost importance to one's heath, leaving aside everything. It is said that "if wealth is lost nothing is lost but if health is lost everything is lost". Because if there is no body, there is nothing can be made available to the individual. Therefore a wise person should make special efforts for achieving this objective. Remember maintainance of health is in your hand and do not expect to happen miracle.

This is possible by promoting rejuvenation, healing, and regeneration of living tissue in the body with the help of this Rasayana therapy. The classical

*Ayurvedic* text says that medicine therapy is divided into prophylactic (preventive) and therapeutic (curative) therapy. Rasayana therapy is included into preventive therapy which is furhter divided into Kuti Praveshika or Indoor-Patient Department and Vatatapika or Outdoor-Patient Department. This unique class of Rasayana therapy enhances the life span, delays aging, improves the intelligence and memory power, promotes health, provides youthful states of the body, betters the body lustier and voice improves the efficiency of the different cognitive abilities and enhances the innate health. It cures diseases how ever deep seated they are. It also reverses the disease process and prevents the re-occurrence. Rasayana replenish the vital fluids of our body, thus keeping us away from life threating diseases.

Everybody knows that aging and death both are natural phenomenon and Acharya Charak considers them inevitable or incurable. No one is immortal. Who so ever born with physical body on this planet has to go one day. There is no exception. But certainly we can extend our life in diseasefree state by taking appropriate steps. Acharya Charak mentions that aging over top most amongst the diseases which can not be cured but the patient be kept free by proper treatment. Acharya Chakrapani mentions that ordinary treatment has got no effect on aging, but Rasayana Therapy particularly Kuti Praveshika is highly effective against aging. It has been mentioned in Charak Samhita that old saint Chyavan became young after the use of Rasayana. Similarly in Vedic literature references of rejuvenation of several rishes are found. In this way premature aging can be treated by Rasayana therapy. However, one should bear in mind that Rasayana is not the final answer to the problem but definitely it can delay the aging process for some time.

**Rasayana Therapy**

Rasayana is one of the eight clinical specialties of *Ayurveda*. Rasayana replenish the vital fluids of our body, thus keeping us away from diseases. The Rasayana therapy enhance the qualities of rasa, enriches it with nutrients so one can attains longevity, memory, intelligence, freedom from disorder, youthfulness, excellence of luster, complexion and voice, optimum development of physique and sense organs, mastery over phonetics and brilliance. Taking Rasayana is helpful to increase the immunity of the person to keep him away from disease and also reverses the disease process and prevents the re-occurrence. The Rasayana are rejuvenators, nutritional supplements and possess strong antioxidant activity.

Taking Rasayana is helpful to increase the immunity of the person to keep him away from disease and also reverses the disease process and prevents the re-occurrence. The Rasayana are rejuvenators, nutritional supplements and possess strong antioxidant activity. With the help of Rasayana therpy our sages/ rishis lived for thousands of years in disease free state.

## Ayurvedic Concept of Aging

Charak has mentioned that growth period is only up to 30 years after that growth stops and aging start to continue. It has been mentioned that each particular thing (organ) is being lost after passing the each decade of life; from early childhood, first three decades, there is incremental growth. After that body start losing some dhatus. This process goes on till death. At the end of sixth, seventh, eighth, ninth and tenth decades of life, remaining functions of motor special senses are lost, respectively.

It is apparent from the preceding that aging is slow and continuous process, which affects various bodily parts at different time. In this way the process of aging definitely begins in the fourth decade of life.

## Modern Concept of Aging and Their Control

According to latest concept of Modern medicine, aging occurs because of malfunctioning of DNA repair mechanism and if we could reverse this action by any means, it will slow down the process of aging. Aging is like cancer and many neurological disorders occur due to damaged DNA.

Though damage of DNA in cells is a continuous phenomenon in our body, but cells keep them repairing. But aging retards such a capacity. The accumulated DNA damage in the body results in wrong kinds of signals (mRNA) as result wrong proteins is being synthesized, which will lead into cell death because of accumulating of toxic substances eventually cell dies. The repair of DNA involves many enzymes; out of this DNA polymerse is of prime importance. The malfunction this enzyme causes aging in brain neurons. Somehow correction in this defect may give chance that DNA repair can be resurrected. Allopathic medicine research indicates that for the damage of DNA, free radicals are the real culprit which are produced during oxidation of food we eat. To neutralize these free radicals vitamin A, vitamin E etc. are used. These compounds are called antioxidants. So, use of antioxidants is the master key to this universal problem. Environmental pollution, irregular habit, junk food, processed food etc. are significant contributor of aging. Symptoms of aging grey hair, wrinkles, loss of sleep, impairment of sight and hearing; brital bones (osteoporosis, arthritis, stiffness, weakened spine). Other sign of aging incluses pain, giddiness, Parkinson's disease, heart, arteries and blood pressure problem, decrased mental function.

We all know that prevention is better than cure. We prevent to rebuild our car engines by changing the engine oil at every 3000 miles; much cheaper. Similarly our medical system is full of expensive high priced "fixes". (Open heart surgery, heart bypass), which can be saved by simple health practices (good health) will prevent heart attacks.

# CHAPTER 2

## Antioxidant Therapy

---

Sunlight is more powerful than any drug; it is safe, effective, and available free of charge. If it could be patented, it would be hyped as the greatest medical breakthrough in history. It's that good.

Mike Adams

All living creatures viz; animals, plants etc require a source of carbohydrates, fats, proteins, minerals, vitamins, water etc. in order to survive and multiply. Oxygen is one of the essential component for life. In another words, existence of life on this earth is dependant on existence of oxygen. Our body with the help of atmospheric oxygen metabolize dietary nutrients and get energy for survival. Oxygen is a double edge sword. On one hand oxygen is unavoidable, on other side it becomes a part of highly reactive atom, which is unstable commonly called "free radicals."

### What are Free Radicals ?

Free radicals are generated by cell's mitochondria as a part of cellular respiration. Cell consists of many different kind of molecules, they are in turn composed of atoms and electrons. Electrons are always present in pair. Free radical is any atom or molecule which has an unpaired electron in outer ring. A unpaired electron will always mean that there is an odd number since pairing of electron goes by 2s. Proton have a positive electrical charge. Electron have negative charge. Electrons move around protons. During oxidation of nutrients free radical are formed. Since free radicals contain an unpaired electron, they are very unstable and reach out and capture electrons from other substances in order to neutralize themselves. This initially stabilizes the free radical but generates another in the process. Soon a chain reaction initiates and within few seconds thousands of free radicals are produced at the site of primary reaction. Excess of free radicals eventually demage the cell. This damage of cells continue which ultimately result into malfunctioning of the organ causing demage to cell DNA and other vital organs of the cells which eventually result into diseases or severe disorders. Cell demage caused by free radicals appears to be a major contributor of aging. Free radicals have been associated in the pathogenesis of more than 50 major diseases.

Our body is equipped to manage with some free radicals and infect needs them to function effectively. However, the damage caused by an overload of free radicals over time may become irreversible and lead to certain diseases including arthritis, diabetes, auto-immune diseases, coronary heart disease, liver disease and some cancers such as oral, esophageal, stomach and bowel cancers, and some neurodegenerative diseases. viz; Parkinson, Alzheimer disease. Oxidation can be accelerated by stress, cigarette smoking, tobacco, alcohol, sunlight, pollution and other factors. These factors are called carcinogens. The term "carcinogen" denotes a chemical substance or a mixture of chemical substances which induce cancer or increase its incidence.

## Antioxidants Anti-aging Compounds

Antioxidants are nutrients present in food that neutralize chemicals called free radicals and protect our cells from damage from them. Plant foods such as colourful fruits and vegetables, nuts and whole grains are rich sources of antioxidants.

Antioxidants are found in certain foods and may prevent some of the damage caused by free radicals by neutralizing them. These include the nutrient antioxidants, vitamins A, C and E, and the minerals copper, zinc and selenium.

The dietary food compounds, such as the phytochemicals in plants, are believed to be superior and have greater antioxidant effects than either vitamins or minerals. These are called the non-nutrient antioxidants and include phytochemicals, such as lycopene in tomatoes and anthocyanin found in cranberries, beta carotene in sweet potato.

## Sources of Antioxidants

Fresh fruits and vegetables are reservoir of antioxidants. Antioxidants are abundant in nuts, grains, and some meats, poultry, and fish. The list of common antioxidants and their sorces are given in Table 2.1

## Table 2.1 Antioxidants and Their Sources

| Antioxidants | Sources |
|---|---|
| Beta carotene | Pumpkin, carrots, bell peppers, spinach, lettuce, sweet potatoes, sqash, apricots, cantaloupe, kale and mangos, winter sqash |
| Lutein | Spinch, green, leafy vegetables such as collard greens, and kale. |
| Catechin | Apples, beans, tea, black or green |
| Anthrocyanins | Beets, eggplant |
| Lycopene | Papaya, guava, watermelon, apricots, pink grapefruit, blood oranges, and other foods, tomatoes and tomato products. |
| Resveratrol | Peanuts |
| Zea xanthin | Basil |
| Flavonoids | Apples, blackberries, blueberries, citrus fruits, grapes and pears. |
| Carotinoids | Apples, apricoat, banana, mango cherries, kiwi fruits, melon and lemon. |
| Vitamin A | Sweet potatoes, carrots, milk, egg yolks, and mozzarella cheese lettuce, |
| Vitamin C (Ascorbic acid) | Water soluble vitamin Oranges, tomatoes, peas, papaya, kale, yellow bell peppears, broccoli, staw berries, cod liver oil, mango, whole milk, kale, dried basil, turnip green peaches, watermelon, sweet potatoes |

| Vitamin E (d Alpha tocophenol) | Fat soluble vitamin. Tofu, spinach, almonds, coconut oil, red pepper, rice bran oil, hazel nut, wheat germ, safflower, corn, and soybean oils, nuts, broccoli, liver, avacardo, shrimp oilve oil |
|---|---|
| Vitamin D | Sun light |
| Selenium | Brazil nuts, brown rice, garlic, onion, wheat germ, white grains, oat meal oysters, tuna, pork, sun flower, tuna, beef, poultry and fortified breads and other grain products. |
| Zinc | Osters, red meat, poultry, beans, nuts, seafood, whole grains, fortified cereals, dairy products, pork, chicken. |

## Supplements

Supplements are vitamins, minerals, amino acids, herbs, fatty acids, phytochemicals. Supplements cannot replace a good diet. But they can compensate for nutrient deficiencies. Although there is little doubt that antioxidants are more effective when obtained from whole foods, rather than isolated from a food and presented in tablet form or softgel form. It has been conclusively proved that antioxidants are good for health. Varieties of antioxidant supplements are freely available. We don't know what antioxidant supplements should be taken also how many types of antioxidant supplements should be taken? It has been proved that some supplements can actually increase cancer risk. It is interesting to note that at normal concentration found in body vitamin C is antioxidant but at higher concentration are prooxidant and thus harmful.

A well-balanced diet, which includes consuming antioxidants from whole foods, is best. If you insist on taking a supplement, seek supplements that contain all nutrients at the recommended levels. It is always advantageous to include colourful fruits and vegetables in your diet. Taking antioxidants in the form of supplements should be the last priority.

A study examining the effects of vitamin E found that it did not offer the same benefits when taken as a supplement. Vitamin E obtained from wheat germ always giving better protection than obtained from tablet. Also, antioxidant minerals or vitamins can act as pro-oxidants or damaging 'oxidants' if they are consumed at levels significantly above the recommended amounts for. Experts say a diet rich in fruits and vegetables can help you ward off infections like colds and flu. That's because these super foods contain immune-boosting antioxidants.

## Can Antioxidants Prevent Diseases?

There are several antioxidant systems within the body that can nullify the ill effect of the oxidative stress that results from regular metabolic processes. Antioxidants in diet can also cancel out the cell-damaging effects of free radicals. These antioxidant supplements act in addition to the endogenous systems and their lack can cause several ill-consequences of oxidative stress. It is observed that people whose diets are rich in fruits and vegetables show lower cancer rate. This has lead to the theory that these diets contain substances, possibly antioxidants, which protect against the development of cancer. Currently results of intense scientific investigation into this topic could not find any relation between dietary supplementation with extra antioxidants and development of cancer.

It is believed that antioxidants slow down the aging process and prevent heart disease and strokes, but the data available is still inconclusive. Therefore from a public health perspective, it is premature to make any recommendations regarding use of antioxidant supplements. In absence of any conclusive evidence, perhaps the best advice, which comes from several authorities in cancer prevention, is to eat large quantity of fruits or vegetables per day.

There is evidence that some types of vegetables and fruits protect against a number of cancers and other diseases. Large studies have shown that people who took regular antioxidants in fruits and vegetables seemed to have lesser incidence of these diseases. In addition, those who took fewer amounts of antioxidants, or had excessive exposure to pro-oxidants like cigarette smoking etc., had a higher risk of these disorders.

For example, oxidation of low density lipoprotein (LDL) in the blood contributes to heart disease. Those taking Vitamin E supplements had a lower risk of developing heart disease.

The exact amounts of antioxidant supplement and their exact role in preventing diseases, however, could not be determined. This meant that some people did get cancers and other oxidative stress related disorders despite adequate fruits and vegetables and antioxidant consumption.

## Is it Worth to Use Antioxidants in Treatment of Diseases?

Several vital organs like the heart, lungs and the brain are vulnerable to oxidative injury. Brain in particular is highly vulnerable because of its high metabolic rate, content of oxygen, and elevated levels of polyunsaturated lipids. Brain and nervous system alone utilize around 20 % of oxygen inhaled. So more vulnerable to damage by free radicals. To protet vital organs intake of supplements are necessary.

Several antioxidant supplements are available to treat neural injury with oxidative stress. Brain injury may result in damage to parts of the brain after a stroke, Alzheimer's disease, Parkinson's disease, multiple sclerosis and other neurodegenerative disorders. After a stroke for example the brain undergoes reperfusion injury that is mediated by oxidative stress. Antioxidants are also being investigated as possible treatments for neurodegenerative diseases such as Alzheimer's disease, Parkinson's disease, and amyotrophic lateral sclerosis.

## Antioxidant Supplements And Their Detrimental Effects

Eugenol, an antioxidant present in clove oil, also possesses toxic effects, if used at high levels. The absorbation of minerals particularly iron and zinc is prevented from Gastro Intestinal tract in persons who consume large amounts of strong reducing agents as antioxidants. In other words antioxidants if taken in excess in diet or supplements may cause more harm than good.

All oxalic acid, tannins and phytic acid, are high in plant-based diets. Persons who take too much phytic acid from beans, legumes, maize, unleavened whole grain bread develop calcium and iron deficiencies. Similarly oxalic acid is present in cocoa, chocolate, spinach, turnip and rhubarb and tannins are present in cabbage, tea and beans. Excess of these in diet may prevent mineral absorption.

Because vitamin C is water soluble vitamin, toxicity associated with high dose of vitamin C is not a serious issue since these can be excreted rapidly in urine. Very high doses of some lipid soluble antioxidants viz; vitamin A, E may have harmful long-term effects, because being fat soluble there are stored in the body.

Plant based antioxidants like carotenes, phytate, vitamin C, vitamin E etc are more powerful in reducing disease risk. Most of the antioxidant compounds in a typical diet are derived from plant sources and belong to various classes of compounds with a wide variety of physical and chemical properties. Some compounds, such as gallates, have strong antioxidant activity, while others, such as the mono-phenols are weak antioxidants. Experts say a diet rich in fruits and vegetables can guard you against infections like colds and flu. That's because these super foods contain immune-boosting antibodies. Natural antioxidant compound present in red grapes and other plants - called resveratrol- blocks many of the cardiovascular benefits of exercise. What is emerging is a new view that antioxidants are not a answer for everything, and that some degree of oxidant stress may be necessary for the body to work correctly. This pivotal study suggests that reactive oxygen species, generally thought of as causing aging and disease, may be a necessary signal that causes healthy adaptations in response to stresses like exercise. So too much of a good thing (like antioxidants in the diet) may actually be detrimental to our health.

**An Ancient *Ayurveda* Anti-aging Formula**

'Amrit Kalash' is an excellent antiaging formula originally designed by sages thousand of years ago. Research has shown that because of its extra ordinary powerful antioxidant property, Amrit Kalash can indeed slow aging process. Yukie Niwa, a Japanese researcher evaluated more than 500 antioxidants over a period of 30 years. He found that the "Amrit Kalash" an ancient Ayurvedic herbal product was most powerful and effective antioxidant of all those tested. The striking feature of

Amrit Kalash was it has antioxidant capabilities which is at least 25,000 times more powerful than those of vitamins C and E. Amrit Kalash-astounding ambrosia is composed of 44 different herbs and fruits that seem to work synergistically enhancing natural strength of one another's antioxidants. Due to presence of its extraordinary antioxidants, Amrit Kalash also defends against wide variety of chronic disorders including cancer in significant way. It prevents tumour from starting, slows down tumour gowth, and even shrinks tumour. It enhances the capacity of attention and alertness that predictably decline with age. At present this amrit kalash is marketed by Maharishi *Ayurveda*.

## Antioxidants: General recommendations

Scientists are divided over whether or not antioxidant supplements offer the same health benefits as antioxidants in foods. It is recommended that people should eat a wide variety of fresh fruits, vegetables, whole grains, lean meats and dairy products every day. Our diet should include five daily serves of fruit and vegetables. One serve is a medium-sized piece of fruit or a half-cup of cooked vegetables. It is also thought that antioxidants and other protective constituents from vegetables, legumes and fruit need to be consumed regularly from early life to be effective. One should cultivate a habit of consuming colourful fresh fruits and vegetables. The colours of fruits and vegetables are clues about type of nutrients they provide. Instead of relying upon supplements, it is always better to obtain antioxidants from food.

# CHAPTER 3

## Rasayana Therapy: For Longevity and Rejuvenation

Due to purification of the body, the capacity of digestion and metabolism is enhanced normal health is restored, all sense organs start working with vigour, old age is prevented and diseases are cured.

Ca. Su.16.17/19

*Rasayana* Therapy is one of the eight branches of *Ayurveda*. Rasayana is a Sanskrit word. Literally 'Rasa' means that which nourishes the body i.e. ahara rasa (food essence) and boosts immunity. Ayana is the method by which rasa is carried to the tissues for biochemical biosynthesis. The quality and quantity (state) of rasa in the body directly governs the state of health of an individual. This body fluid of good quality should not only be present in adequate quantity but also it should be of high quality and able to circulate throughout the entire cells of the body to provide the type of nourishment they need. This is essential for healthy state of living. The aim of Rasayana therapy is to boost normal functioning of the enzymes that are present in the tissue cells. It is also called rejuvenation therapy. This branch of Ashtang *Ayurveda* aims at achieving a long and healthy life. In Charak Samhita, Rasayana listed at seventh of the eight divisions of *Ayurveda*.

Rasayana therapy has unimaginable and astonishing effects. According to Acharya Charak a person undergoing Rasayana therapy attains:

❖ "It preserves our vital energy so that they can increase to the point at which they can bring about an inner transformation.

❖ Rasayana therapy strives to improve our physical, mental and ethical qualities.

❖ It restores youthfulness and improves complexion, memory power, will power, body strength, luster, sweetness of voice; increase physical strength and immunity, cures drowsiness, laziness and weakness.

❖ It maintains correct balance of tridoshas.

❖ It strengthens memory and intelligence, gives happiness and promotes life that is beneficial to others, promotes longevity and retards the aging process.

❖ Rasayana are aimed at nourishing sapta dhatu of human body (blood, lymph, bone marrow, bone, flesh, adipose tissues and semen) and prevents degenerative changes and illness. Most of these Rasayana may be consumed regularly as food for maintaining balanced mental and physical health.

❖ As Rasayana nourish blood, lymph and bone marrow, three major organ systems that regulate production, differentiation and functioning of immune cells, it was speculated that Rasayanas may modulate immune system favourably for patients.

❖ Rasayana which has marked action on reproductive organs and also nourishes shukra dhatu.

❖ Helps to attain optimal strength and sharpness of sense organs.

❖ Rasayana invigorates the body in general by sustaining the balance between anabolism and catabolism

❖ Rasayana therapy keeps the body and mind pleasant.

❖ Prevents wasting of muscles, delays aging process, keep strong bones, tendons etc. prevents osteoporosis, improves whole body circulation, prevents graying of hair and provide good sleep and appetite."

(Charak Samhita)

It is widely agreed that the best herbs to use for overall wellness are the anti-stress immune competence enhancing adaptogens, according to experts around the world from all traditions and walks of life. Though in *Ayurveda* the concept is thousands of years old, western bioscience also has recently discovered adaptogens, known in *Ayurveda* as the Rasayana and in traditional Chinese medicine as the superior herbs. At present an adaptogens must have following properties.

1. Produces a nonspecific response; for instance, an increase in the power of resistance against multiple (physical, chemical or biological) stressors.
2. Has a normalizing influence, irrespective of the direction of change from physiological norms caused by the stressor. (This is the principle of a medicinal substance that is "two-directional")
3. Is innocuous and does not influence normal body functions more than required

Today western scientist found, which were confirming what thousands of years of traditional Ayurvedic Medicine told them: Ashwagandha and Tulsi specifically are two of the premier adaptogens known, and that the Rasayanas of *Ayurveda* in general are all adaptogens

Amongst the most researched and esteemed anti-stress immuno-enhancing adaptogens are:

| Amalaki (*Emblica officinalis*) | Ashwagandha(*Withania somnifera*) |
| Guduchi (*Tinospora cordifolia*) | Haritaki (*Terminalia chebula*) |
| Long Pepper (*Piper longum*) | Brahmi (*Bacopa monniera*) |
| Shatavari (*Asparagus racemosus*) | Basil (*Ocimum sanctum*) |

## Classification of Rasayana

Acharya Sushruta has classified Rasayana into three broad categories

## 1. Based on State of Health

This group includes Rasayana which promote vitality and longevity; mental function and strength and vigour e.g. triphala, haritaki brahmi, amalaki etc.

This group of Rasayana is discussed in coming chapter 6 to 33.

## 2. Based on Diet and Lifestyle

This group includes diet and Lifestyle of individual e.g. milk, honey, ghee, almond, Fig, Dates etc. This group of Rasayana is discussed in chapter 4, 34 and 35.

## 3. Based on Place of Therapy

There are two types of Rasayana chikitsa based on place of therapy

1.  Kuti Praveshhika Rasayana: Indoor Rasayana Therapy
2.  Vatatapika Rasayana: Outdoor Rasayana Therapy.

## 1. Kuti Praveshhika Rasayana

This procedure is also called "Kaya kalpa" (total renovation of the body.) In comparision to Vatatapica method, this procedure is more complicated. It requires patient's determination and full trust in procedure he is going to undertake. After finishing required purification programme viz; complete package of Purvakarma i.e. oleation, swedan, snehan and Panchakarma i.e. vaman, virechan, basti, on an auspicious day patient enters the Kuti (room)specially designed for rejuvenation. The patient is required to stay in the same room up to three months. The room should possibly be outside city in pollution free area close to the nature. Sufficient care is taken not to expose patient in direct sun light, wind, cold etc. Patient is kept under controlled conditions in air-conditioned to eliminate variation in climate. All adequate medicines and amenities required for daily life should be made available in the room.

The patient is kept under medical observation of an *Ayurvedic* specialist preferably trained in rejuvention. During the course of the entire treatment he is not permitted to contact outside world. It is mendatory for the patient to remain in positive frame of mind and emotion. To maintain tranquility of mind, he should do yogasan, pranayam and meditation. During this treatment, he/she is provided sattvic Ayurvedic diet considering the age, sex, status of health, constitution; he/she is not permitted to bring food from outside. The patient is advised to remain in relaxed condition. He is given daily whole body massage with medicated oil. A complete regime of Rasayana is given to the patient one by one. After completion of the full course of treatment, the arteries become soft and smooth, the constitution of blood changes, clots get dissolved and new cells are formed. After successful completion of entire procedure, when he or she comes out of the kuti, the body is completely rejuvenated. All the old *dhatu* (body tissues) are replaced by new, energetic and lively *dhatu*. The person acquires all the benefits of Rasayana therapy. He will become youthful, with full of enegy, vigour and will be disease free. In short he will be a all together different person. Unfortunately inspite of tremendoyus advantages of this therapy, it is not popular. There are very few persons who know this therapy and very few centres where this type of treatment is available.

## 2. Vatatapika Rasayana

This type of Rasayana therapy is prescribed to a patient, who does not have time, money and enthusiasm or one who cannot undergo the full length of the treatment for some valid reason. The patient undergoing this therapy receives a short package of *Rasayana therapy*. Patient is allowed to continue his daily routine simultaneously. The patient is advised dietary changes and changes in lifestyle in addition to possible Rasayana medicines. These medicines are carefully chosen considering the patient's age, sex, *prakruti* (constitution), habits, living conditions and diseases acquired in the past and present status of the body. We can say that this is a outdoor trement. This type is less beneficial than Kuti Praveshhika but because of its convenience, people prefer it. At present majority of patients opt for this type of treatment. However to get best benefits out of this theratpy patient is advised not to consume oily, sour, spicy, fatty food during the course of treatment. Patient is not allowed to drink alcohol or smoke. Any one Rasayana suggested in Charak *Samhita* can be used.

Charak and Sushrutra have given number of formulations of Classical Rasayana. Some examples of Classical formulations are Amrit Rasayana, Brahma Rasayana, Laxami Vilas Ras, Laxman Vilas Ras, Makrdhawaj vati, Navjeevan Ras, Shukar Amrit Vati, Smritisagar Ras, Suvarn Malini Vasant, Suvarn Vasant Malti etc.

These classical Rasayana formulae, contain a large number of ingredients, including minerals, pearl, coral and gems, and include a specially processed mercury (the word ras indicates mercury as an ingredient). Because of negative publicity and high cost, the use of the classical Rasayana formulas has declined considerably, and most of the preparations available now have herbal ingredients with a couple of mineral and animal products. The non-availability and wild life protection act has made the use of musk, amber, and parts of wild-life animals nearly impossible.

The current Rasayana formulas are based on such ingredients as Emblica officinalis, Terminalia belerica, Terminalia chebula, Shilajit (a mineral exudate high in fulvic acid), Long pepper, Black pepper, Ginger, processed Guggul, Guduchi, Ashwagandha, Shatavari and similar ingredients.

There is no other class of nutritional or herbal support can offer more health prevention than adaptogens. They are powerful tonic herbs with the ability to restore and rebalance health. No other botanicals can offer as many health promoting, stress boosting and body balancing benefits. Adaptogens supports the integrated regulation of our body systems, especially the endocrine, immune, and nervous systems. This helps to modulate our stress response keeping us cool under fire and more balanced in an increasingly unbalanced world irrespective of source of stress. Adaptogens are very special plants with exceptional qualities. These plants mostly grow in the mostly extreme and inhospitable environments around the world. Their ability to survive and thrive make them special. Some of them are holy basil, licorice, ashwagandha, ginseng.

Rasayana has meanings beyond healthful substances. Rasayana Shastra in Ancient India was much less developed than today. Nevertheless, the use and practice of Rasayana was widespread in Ancient India, and some examples of applied Rasayana include paints used in the caves of Ajanta and Ellora, Maharashtra state, the steel of Vishnustambha (literal meaning: the tower of Vishnu), and a processed wood sample in the Kondivade caves near the Rajmachi fort in Maharashtra. In all these monuments Rasayana shatra is beautifully depicted.

# CHAPTER 4

## Ayurvedic Diet and Lifestyle

---

**When diet is wrong, medicine is of no use. When diet is correct medicine is of no need.**

Ayurvedic proverb

*Ayurveda* is a very vast and ancient Indian medical healing science. There are many diseases for which there are no cures in modern science. The approach of modern medicines is to suppress the symptoms of disease by number of drugs. The disease remains in the body, which result into continuous attack on immune system of the body resulting in many dreadful diseases. Realizing this fact, more and more people in the world are switching over to alternative system of healing which includes massage, panchakarma, herbal and diet regimens, and change in lifestyle. We are capable of taking charge our own healing. Ailment like rheumatic pain, backache, and stiff neck, are relieved for a long period by appropriate Panchakarma therapy. Western medicines prescribe anti-inflammatory drugs, pain killers, and antibiotics etc. which are manmade (synthetic) and majority with very serious side effects. Allopathy system of medicine is a symptom based medicine branch which addesses only symptoms, actual disease remains in the body. Migraine, which has no effective solution in modern medicines, is relieved for a sustained period by shirodhara technique. Western medicines have no answer for illness affecting metabolism, psychosomatic diseases, asthma, rheumatoid arthritis, ulcerative colitis, scabies, psoriasis, neurological diseases, auto immune diseases etc. *Ayurveda* is the science of how to live in harmony with our bodies and our planet. How to eat is considered major therapeutic tool, one of the most important things you can do to help yourself in Ayurvedic perceptive.

## A. Ayurvedic Diet

*Ayurveda* is the highly accurate and personalized method of treatment. Before commencing the actual treatment, it analyzes one's constitution and type of illness. Accordingly, it prescribes gentle, natural and effective therapies includes system of medicines that focuses on preventing illness, panchakarma, Rasayana therapy etc. Unlike other medical sciences, *Ayurveda* instead of focusing on treatment of any particular disease, it focuses more on the healthy living and well being. For healthy living, it focuses on consuming right kind of healthy and nutritious diet. Depending upon disease, Ayurvedic doctor puts several restriction on diet.

In *Ayurveda*, food is considered not only as source of the basic ingredients like proteins, fats, carbohydrates, minerals and vitamins but something which serves as a source of energy for mind and soul. At present people are careless about their food. Our eating habit has changed drastically over a period of time. Rather than taking food at home, we prefer to eat food outside in reastaurant seeing only its presentation and taste. Food prepared at home perhaps may not match in appearance and taste but one thing is certain that it is nutritious and hygienic and sattvic and will provide energy not only to your body but will also to your mind and soul.

You are what you eat. What you eat affects your health. When you do not watch your diet, your health faces problems. Right diet is the principal factor in the treatment of the physical body that is built up by food. Without changing the diet, it is next to impossible to make fundamental change in our body. By correcting the diet, we may eliminate causes of the diseases. *Ayurveda* emphasizes the correct diet for each individual on the basis of health.

Food is fuel that makes us function, that gives energy, builds body and repairs it. In order to remain healthy we should go for ayurvdic diet. An ayurvedic diet makes generous use of full spectrum of fresh vege tables, fruits, grains, legumes and milk. It plays with herbs and spices, often kitchen items like fresh ginger, cardamom, cinnamon, turmeric, cumin, coriander, clove, fennel, ajwain etc. are used to support agni, the digestive fire within us. An Ayurvedic food not only affect our body but also is considered to affect mind as well as body. By understanding how to prepare food best suited to our mind and bodies, we can utilize nutrition as deeper source of healing. Our diets are largely under own control, no one else can eat for us.

Once the concepts of cooking fresh light vegetarian meals in an Ayurvedic way are grasped practically speed with which you can heal and balance can be tremendously encouraging. But Ayurvedic cuisine can encompass a wide variety of all sort of vegetarian dishes so long as they remain fresh, easy to digest, not fermented and prepared with loving care. It is important to understand that *Ayurveda* is a healing science.

## Ayurvedic Diet and Nutrition

The *Ayurveda* has a different vision of diet and nutrition. The primary concern of *Ayurveda* is your ability to digest the food. The second is to eat foods befitting to your constitution. *Ayurveda* does not distinguish between food and medicine, *Ayureda* gives equal weightage to both. It is believed that wrong food, the absence of nutritive food or diet are responsible for causing disease in the body. This can only be corrected with appropriate food. Here food becomes the medicine to heal the body of its ailment.

*Ayurvedic* diet is assimilated into the body and contributes to its nourishment for body and mind. This transformation of 'food' into nutrition is mediated by 'jathragni' or fire, which forms the edifice upon which the Ayurvedic system is built.

*Ayurveda* says that most of the common ailments are a result of poor nutrition. *Ayurvedic* nutrition is concerned importantly with the dietary requirements of individuals. Any anomaly in the body is thought to originate in the digestive system, and therefore it become crucial not to ignore even minor digestive complaints, as it could be indicative of a disease. Remember the more we depart from nature in our living habits the more we may suffer in long run. Most diseases are due to our incorrect diet. The cure for such wrong eating is not in better drug.

Spices and herbs form an integral part of Ayurvedic healing, mainly because of its power to be easily absorbed in the body. On the one hand, it boosts the digestive capacity of the body and on the other, it flush out toxins from the body, ensuring the cells in the body to obtain right nutrition from the diet.

## Harmful Foods That Hasten Aging

In order to increase life span it is essential to know the foods that hasten aging. If we eat food such as bread, cereals and sugar in the refined state as white bread, white sugar and polished rice, they produce more acids in the body, which in turn change the pH of the body. This will result into development of disease. If we consume in the natural state as natural brown sugar, as whole wheat bread and as natural brown rice they are safe.

## 1. Wheat

Wheat is principal source of energy and nutrition, and used through out the world for making bread. Wheat is grind to flour before use as food. Until recently, wheat grains were crushed between two large horizontal stones. This method preserve all parts of karnel and the product was called whole wheat. If it is finely ground, it is called whole wheat flour. Still in town and villeges you will find this technique of crushing wheat. The value of stone grinding is that however grain is grind slowly, the advantages that it remains unheated, nutrients are preserved, and a whole food is obtained. Currently, steel roller mills have superseded stone grinding, same is true for domestic flour mill. The technology has changed. The good thing is that this mill grind grain at much faster rate but they remove the precious wheatgerm the flour, resulting colossal loss of vitamins and minerals in the refining process. By doing so we unknowningly remove the very life of the wheat because locked in the wheat germ is an oil, which is man's greatest food. Wheat germ oil contains important essential vitamin E, lack of this vitamin also led to heart attack. For vegetarian people wheat is the principal source of vitamin E. unfortunately in modern grinding valuable vitamin E is destroyed.

## 2. Cane Sugar

Sugar is the most common carbohydrate used all over the world. Among diffferent types of carbohydrates, sucrose or cane sugar, fructose or grape sugar, levulose or fruit sugar and lactose of milk sugar are used considerably in our diet. Cane sugar also called white sugar is produced in large quantaties. It is derived commercially from sugarcane and beat root. Cane sugar because of its low cost and easy availability, widely consumed by the public. This cane sugar once enter in our body, it slowly converted into levulose and dextrose, so that it can be utilized by our body. Like starch, it must undergo a digestive process. In case of starch digestion begin in mouth, but it is delayed until sugar reaches the intestine.

Now a days with changes in food habit, consumption of sugar has increased at alarming rate, all over the world, which has resulted into increase in incidence of several diseases. Medical science have undoughtably proved that white sugar is extremely injurious to our health and it is doing more harm than good. The heat and chemical process employed in sugar refinery kills vitamin and separates mineral elements, protein etc from sap leaving nothing but pure sugar crystals. Excess sugar can cause hypoglycemia and diabetes.

## 3. Common Salt

Salt is needed for working of nerves and muscles of our body. It can prevent catarrh, assists in production of hydrochloric acid in the stomch. Thus a certain amount of salt is essential for life. Our body require salt in very small amounts. Our requirement of salt ranging from 10-15 g daily depending upon climate and occupation of the person. However many people use excess of salt. Consumption of extra salt puts extra burden on kidney and in many cases this may result into high blood pressure, swelling of the legs and ankles, create artificial thrist. So a person drinks enormous quantities of water which will be deoposited in the body leads to obesity in due course. Extra salt is injurious to health, may develop stomach ulcer, stomach cancer, hardening of arteries and heart disease.

Food rich in common salt includes pickles, papads, meat, fish, salted nuts, biscuits, chicken, eggs, cheese, dried fruits, carrot and radish should be avoided. However there is no harm in taking low sodium foods like cereals, sugar, honey, fresh fruits, cabbage, brinjal, cauliflower, potato, tomato, peas etc.

## 4. Hot Beverages

In recent times consumption of hot beverages viz; tea and coffee increased at alarming rate all over the world. Tea contains caffeine (2.5-5.0%), tannin (7-14%), coffee contains more caffeine than tea. During boiling, caffeine comes out quickly followed by tannin. Because of high contents of caffeine and tannin, tea and coffee are taken for their stimulating effect, they remove feeling of tiredness and provide freshness after drinking. In long run this will culminate into habit. Tea can not be given status of food. It slows down digestion. Consumption of tea and coffee both are detrimental to health. Aggressive marketing by the companies compel us to drnk tea/coffee.

## Types of Food

Diet is considered to be vital for a human body as it provides the basic nutrients. These are necessary to carry out the fundamental activities of digestion and metabolism. *Ayurveda* has categorized food into three types based on its basic quality *viz;* Sattvik, Rajasic and Tamasic.

Trigun or three guns sattva, rajas and tamas are the three main components of the mind. The mental powers exist parallel to tridoshas *(vata, pitta* and *kapha).* These three gunas determines one's nature, belief and perception on the basis of his psychology and body constitution.

## Table4.1 Relationship of Diet and Individual's Characters

| Type of diet | Individual's Characters |
|---|---|
| **A Sattvic Diet**<br>❖ Sattvic diet, purest diet, nourishes the body, calms and purifies the mind,<br>❖ Sattvic food includes cereals, whole wheat bread, fresh fruits, vegetables, pure fresh juices, milk, butter, cheese, legumes, nuts, sprouted seeds & whole grains, spices, natural sweeteners, herbal teas and oils. Sattvic food includes balance of all six tastes. | **1.  Sattvic Person**<br>Pure, Conciousness; Very intelligent; Sharp memory; Promote knowledge by reasonable means; Polite; Unselfish; Control over mind and speech; Cheerful; Calm, and Quite; Full faith in God; Reacts to Pain and Pleasure properly; Alert; Strong Will Power |
| **B Rajasic diet**<br>❖ Rajasic diet hot, bitter, sour, dry or salty, not palatable; destroy the mind-body equilibrium, over stimulate the body and making the mind restless and uncontrollable.<br>❖ Rajsic foods include hot substances, such as sharp spices or strong herbs, stimulants such as coffee and teas, fish, eggs, salt and chocolate etc. They include most of fermented foods including yoghurt, garlic, pepper of all kind, eggs, cheese, white sugar, most sweetners, beans, avocado, radishes, citrus, peanut etc. | **2. Rajasic Person**<br>Acquire knowledge by any way; Average intelligent; Average memory ;Over ambitious; Strong desire for status and wealth; Selfish, Dynamic; Questions God; Sometimes Rude and Angry; Brave; Cruel and Greedy, Follow Health Advise if convinced, Over reacts to Pain and Pleasure; Hyper active, Fluctuating Will Power |

| C Tamasic Diet | 3. Tamasic Person |
|---|---|
| ❖ Tamasic diet benefits neither the mind nor the body. Prana (life force) or energy is withdrawn, powers of reasoning become clouded and a sense of inertia sets in.. The body's resistance to disease is destroyed and the mind gets filled with dark emotions, such as anger and greed.<br><br>❖ Tamasic food includes most fast food, fried food, frozen food, microwaved food, processed food, leftover night food, meat, drugs, chemicals, mushrooms, lard, poultry, alcohol, tobacco, onions, garlic, fermented foods such as vinegar, over ripe substances. | Ignorant about Knowledge; Non Intelligent, Poor memory; Lethargic; Selfish, No desire for Anything; No control in Body; Depressed; Fearfull, Believes in Untruth, Ignorant about Health; Does not follow Medical Advice; Fail to react Pain and Pleasure, Lazy; No Interest, Limited Will Power. |

As per our ancient science, these three qualities of sattva (purity), rajas (activity, passion, the process of change) and tamas (darkness) exist together in equilibrium. In the manifestation of any project, we need sattva to design the plan, rajas to reorganize and initiate its physical manifestation and tamas to complete it. The strength of each of these qualities differs from person to person. By managing our intake of foods that induce these qualities in us, we can modify, regulate and control our actions, thoughts and even our expressions to some extent. Just like by choosing the unadulterated gas we can improve and lengthen the life of our car, by using our understanding in choosing our food we can improve the quality of our lives. It is the state of mind which is responsive for the onset of any disease.

The first step in commencing Ayurvedic diet is to eat a primarily sattvic diet avoiding rajasic and tamsic diet. In other word you begin to eat food which are fresher and pure. This means foods free from additives, preservatives, and pesticides as much as possible. In another words organic food should be our preference. Once you are getting used to it, you can begin to consider some of the subtler points of Ayurvedic food dynemics. A food taste (rasa) is important. Each of these six tastes has different effects on the body. A food has varying impacts on the body, from the time you first taste it(rasa) to the time it enters your stomach (virya), to the time it has been absorbed (vipak).

## Properties of Food

Like all herbs and medicinal plants, all food is composed of three basic factors. These are 1. five great elements i.e. panchamahabhutas 2. six tastes and 3. twenty attributes.

**Table 4.2 Properties of Food.**

| Five Elements | Akash, Air, Fire, Water and Earth, |
|---|---|
| Six Tastes | Sweet, Sour, Salty, Bitter, Pungent Astringent |
| Twenty Attributes | Heavy, Slow, Cold, Wet, Sticky, Dance Soft, Firm, Subtle, and clear and their opposite. |

Food which we consumed is made up of panchamahabhutas. Different combination of these panchamahabhutas confers different qualities to foods. One of the most important of such qualities is that of rasa which may be one of the following six tastes i.e. sweet, sour, salty, pungent, bitter and astringent or a mixture of these. The predominance of water results into sweet taste; a higher concentration of earth and fire leads to sour taste ; the predominance of air and akash provide a bitter taste; excess of air and fire lead to pungent taste; and air and earth render as astringent taste to food. All the important nutrients that we need for life, such as fats, proteins, carbohydrates, minerals, vitamins etc. are contained in meal that consists six tastes. Relation of panchmahabhutas with taste, constitution i.e. *vata, pitta* and *kapha*, and senses are depicted in Table 4.3.

**Table 4.3 Relation of Panchamahabhutas Taste, Constitution and Senses**

| Elements | Taste | Constitution | Senses |
|---|---|---|---|
| Eather(Akash) | Bitter | *Vata* | Hearing |
| Air | Bitter Astringent Pungent | *Vata* | Touch |

| Fire (Tejas) | Pungent<br>Sour<br>Salty | *Pitta* | Sight |
| Wate(Jala) | Salty<br>Sweet | *Kapha*<br>*Pitta* | Taste |
| Earth | Sweet<br>Sour<br>Astringent | *Kapha* | Smell |

## Digestive Power (Agnis or Enzymes)

According to *Ayurveda* proper diet and digestion are one of the principal pillars of health. An improper diet and inadequate digestive capacity results in undigested material in the body, leading to the production of *ama,* a toxic material that blocks the channels of the body and initiates disease processes. The digestive power or jatharagni of individual is dependent upon balance of doshas in body. Any imbalance in doshas leads to disorder of digestion and metabolism in the body. Good digestion nourishes the body. The food contain agni is called jatharagni. But without prana nothing can happen. Our food contains solar energy which can only be utilized in the body through digestion. Eating the proper foods will make a big difference in your wellbeing. There are two aspects to the food and nutrition. One is the physical food you eat, digest, and assimilate. In this process, the organs of your digestive system have a big role. The second aspect of it is what you consume through your mind-body. What you see, hear, taste, smell, feel, and think are all important for your wellbeing and impact your health considerably. For example, stress plays a key role in the health. Charak had recognized the importance of the environment in the total health. Remember, everything in your environment is composed of doshas that interact with your own doshas. You are affected by everything else which goes on in this universe as you are part and parcel of this cosmos.

Agni helps various tissues of the body to produce secretions, metabolic reactions, and other processes needed to create energy and maintain and repair the body. Agni is also part of the immune system since its heat destroys harmful organisms and toxins. The activity of agni varies throughout the day and maintaining the strength and natural flow of your digestive fires is needed for good digestion, good immune function, and resistance to disease. Agni is needed to form ojas. Many diseases are due to poor digestion.

## Tips for healthy living

If you want to remain healthy and active for a long time, here are some very important recommendations, which are if followed, will keep you hale and hearty and you will enjoy long disease free life.

1. As per, vitiated saptadhatus, abnormal doshas, and malas, obstruction or blockage of different channels, weakened jatharagni and presence of *ama* are the five possible causes of all diseases.
2. You should select food items that suit your prakruti and benefit your health. Remember everybody is unique in constitution so what suits someone else may not suit you. You will have to find out what suits you and stick to it.
3. Food should contain oily or fatty contents in proper proportions. Fatty content will make the food tasty and delicious, promotes secretion of digestive juices, and assist in proper digestion of food. Use only olive oil or rice bran oil in kitchen.
4. Take the food according to the place, timing, climate, own constitution and temperament.
5. Decide the appropriate quantity of food based upon your constitution, weight, strength of your jatharagni and current season.
6. Keep off too much dry food like packaged, caned and junk food.
7. One should not consume, iced water or ice-cream after meals, as it slows Agni and digestion; therefore ice cold water is poison and hot water is nectar.
8. Avoid white wheat flour, white sugar and salt.
9. Avoid food containing preservative, artificial sweetener, flavour, colour, taste enhancer etc.
10. Eat less, chew more. Skip high caloric deserts. Opt for more fresh fruits and vegetables..

## B. Lifestyle

Today modern science has given us everything. The most ignored concept of modern science is health and lifestyle. Today with the introduction of vaccination, development of new generation of antibiotics and synthetic drugs; better medical facilities and awareness about health and hygiene, we has almost eliminated the threat from most infectious diseases viz; typhoid, cholera, tuberculosis etc. As a result death due to these diseases is considerably reduced. But a new type of diseases of modern age called lifestyle diseases are the primary causes of today's concern. They include hyper tension, heart attack, stroke, obesity, diabetes, diseases associated with smoking, and alcohol, drug abuse, tobacco induced cancer, autoimmune diseases, chronic bronchitis, emphysema and premature mortality. It is true that nobody in this world is immortal. Everybody has to die of something at some time, but lifestyle diseases take people at relatively early age. Heart attack and cardiac arrest, stroke and cancer have become routine phenomenon in our society.

Today we find little time for entertainment, social life, exercise, regular eating and adequate sleeping. Everybody is in mad race for money. Personnel priorities are given least importance, while corporate interests and personal ambitions are center of activity.

They are mainly caused due to sedentary lifestyle, workaholism, irregular sleep pattern, craze for wealth, consumption-based happiness, absence of regular sleep, leisure, socializing, taking of junk food, extended working hours, mental stress, reduced physical activity, smoking and consumption of alcohol etc. Since factors like heredity, sex, surrounding atmosphere, age etc. cannot be avoided but definitely we can manage our own lifestyle to avoid the entry of these dreadful diseases. Lifestyle diseases are potentially preventable, and can be lowered with changes in diet, lifestyle, and environment.

External factors like change in weather and internal factors via; wrong diet, emotions can trigger these imbalances. Rather than analyze and name millions of body parts and diseases Charak Samhita holds that it is happiness and unhappiness that result in health and disease.

Ayurvedic theory states that all imbalances and disease in the body begin with stress in awareness or consciousness of the individual. unhealthy lifestyles, which promote ill health.

Our health is greatly influenced by our Lifestyle. As per our routine plays an important role on our health. A natural life is a life regulated according to the individual constitution. *Ayurveda* is the life science, which tells us about all details of our Lifestyle and dietary habits. According to proper diet and daily routine balance our body doshas and we can live long healthy life without being affected by disease or illness. In today's life it is really hard to follow the instructions and switch to natural healthy diet because from childhood we are used to those tastes which we are using, We need to make up our mind for healthy routine: drink more fluids during the summer, avoid foods that are pungent, acidic or salty, wear light clothes and avoid strenuous exercise.

One should give preference to health in life. Maintenance of good health is in your hand. Also you cannot purchase it. There is no substitute for our right living. As long as you are not living life in harmony with nature, no system of medicine can help you.

## Deep Breathing

Deep breathing freely delivers enough oxygen to each and every cell of the body tissues. But with sallow breathing, enough oxygen is not available; due to lack of pran energy will result into stiffness, depression, congestion. We need to open our respiratory channels through deep breathing.

We should know that it is our expectations, our arrogance, and our inflexibility, which are the primary causes of sorrow in our day to day life. Remember, the fundamental cause of grief does not lie in outer world, but it lies within oneself.

## Anxiety

Our anxiety is often vague and misdirected. Remember it is not always possible for us to change or to avoid the situations of life and therefore we should accept them gracefully without grievances or complaints. More often than not, we allow external situations to affect us. Anxious people imagine worst end result and spend most of time dreading things that may never happen.

Whatever we can do by ourselves to improve our health is effective and beneficial in long run than other person can do for us. Only when we have failed in our attempts, clinical facility should be availed. Remember maintenance of health is our responsibility and our hope that something miraculous will happen or third person will restore your health, then you are mistaken. It is proved that stress is the root cause of many diseases, which need to be addressed to remain healthy.

## Ojas

Qualities of the mind and emotions, such as less anger, inner calm, more positive thoughts, and more feelings of love and compassion are described in the Charak Samhita as qualities that uphold ojas and lessen the risk of heart disease and all illnesses.

Thus the quality of your inner emotions directly determines the quality of your heart health. Be vigilant to prevent negative emotions and thinking from creeping into your inner life. When you make the choice to be positive in emotions and healthy in behavior, a multitude of health benefits will naturally be yours. Ours thoughts can be one of the main causes of our aging process." As we think so shall we become" our thoughts create our reality. By beginning to change our thinking, we can age gracefully.

## Life or Pran

Pran is a term which is used as a very useful step in descriptions of life. The conjuction of body with vital pran is known as life. It is the primary life force the subtle energy of air. It is the master force behind all mind body functions. It is the subtlest form of the breath that pervades the entire human body. It is more than the normal breath and the essence of life. It keeps every tissue of the human body alive and flows throughout the body. Whenever there is obstruction anywhere in the free flow of pran, there is pain. Pain is mainly a manifestation of the obstruction in the free flow of the Pran. This obstruction is caused by bad food habits, abnormal Lifestyles and defective postures. Pran therapy tackles these obstructions and set the flow of pran in the right direction.

*Ayurveda* believes that health is a state of positive attitude. Negative thinking produces stress, shame, anger and fear. These emotions disturb our digestion, metabolism and immune function and age us. Negative thoughts and the feelings are the primordial cause of disease, toxin, deficiencies etc. Autoimmune disease is making us sick today. Our bodies are attacking themselves. Arthritis, cancer, heart disease, MS are caused by defect in immune system. Meditation is a Ayurvedic practice of letting go of world's thoughts and merging with universal mind. Hence by following *Ayurvedic* way of life, we remain in harmony with nature and when we do that nature always give health, happiness and harmony of body, mind and soul. Take control of your health, read books, get second opinion and don't trust some one just because they have a degree. Remember you know better yourself than somebody else.

# CHAPTER 5

## Herbs and Their Role in Human Health

---

**Secret of health both for mind and body is not to mourn for the past, worry about the future, or anticipate trouble but to live in present moment wisely and earnestly.**

Buddha

Before human beings had started practicing agriculture, they were knowing the usefulness of medicinal plants. Herbal medicines are one of the most ancient forms of health care for mankind. History tells that the use of plants for healing purposes has been prevalent around the globe in all cultures of civilization. The traditions of medicinal use of plants, as understood by the earlier generations are passed on to the next generation. In present day situation, this wealth of knowledge about use of plants as a source of medicine is being preserved by traditional physicians and herbal practitioners of different ethnic societies.

The World Health Organization (WHO) has listed over 21,000 species (including synonyms) that have been reported for medicinal uses around the world. Moreover, it estimates that more than 80 % of the world's population even today relies on traditional health care. It was also reported that 30 % or more of modern drugs were derived from plant sources. This shows the importance of plants in present times. India and China are principal and largest users of medicinal plants. China has listed approximately 500 species of plants as official drugs. Around 30 to 60 % medicines consumed account for traditional Chinese herbal products which second most used medical system after Western allopathic system. The current market size of herbs and natural health products in China is US$ 650 milion. In India 60 % of registered physicians are involved in non-allopathic systems of medicine which includes *Ayurveda,* homeopathy, unani etc. The Indian herbal drug market size is about US$ 1 billion. In the last decade the market for herbal products has increased tenfold in United States alone. There is a greater interest in complementary and alternative medicines including herbal medicines. The current potential of herbal medicine is estimated about $ 80-250 biilion in Europe and USA. Herbal medicines alone in US pharmaceuticals constitute a multi billion dollar business. Medicinal plant based drug industries is progressing very fast in India.

It is difficult to give precise definition of medicinal plant. Plants produce wide array of bioactive principles and constitute a rich source of medicines. The herbal products can be isolated and identified as potential for medicines. Herbal medicines are prepared from a variety of plant parts as whole plant, leaves, stems, rhizome, flowers roots, flowers, bark, etc. They usually contain biologically active ingredients and are used primarily for treating mild or chronic ailments. The valueable medicinal properties of different plants are due to the presence of several constituents i.e. saponins, tannins, alkaloids, flavonoids, terpenoids etc. Artemisinin produced by *Artemisia annaua* plant is very effective against *Plasmodium falciparum, P. vivax* and also drug resistant parasite. For 2,000 years powdered root of *Rauvofia serpentina* has been used in treatment of mental illness in india.

In India 15,000 plant species have been identified and out of which 7,000 to 8,500 plants are used by traditional communities for curing various disesaes. It is generally estimated that over 6,000 traditional plants in India are in real commercial use.

Aromatic plants are a special class of plants used for their aroma and flavour. Many of them are exclusively used also for medicinal purposes in aromatherapy as well as in various systems of medicine. Similarly a number of medicinal plants also produce essential oils as well as being used for perfumery e.g. *Petroselinum sativum, Daucus carota, Anethum graveolens* and *Pimpinella anisum* etc.

India being one of the mega biodiversity centers of the world is one of the richest countries in plant wealth due to its wide range of geographical, ecological and biological diversities. The country possesses typical tropical to temperate ecological zones, warm humid to dry hot arid areas apart from cold desert. Accordingly, India has been considered as a treasure house for valuable biotic entities. Many of the plant species are directly or indirectly in use as the sources of raw materials for medicinal and cosmetic industries, the oldest medicinal system in Indian sub-continent. The *Charak Samhita*, an age old (1,000 BC) written document on herbal therapy, reports on the production of about 340 herbal drugs and their indigenous uses. Human being has been in a very old and common relationship in nature. Possibly, early human beings had learnt usefulness of medicinal herbs before they started practicing agriculture.

*Ayurveda* is the science that came into existence since ancient era. *Ayurvedic* classical formulations and single herbs have been tested for thousands of years on people and have proved safe.

## Ayurvedic Herbs

The herbs used in *Ayurveda* are different from each other, in terms of a number of factors. A number of herbs vary according to their taste, while others are categorized according to their medicinal value. There are mainly three different categories of herbs: mild, strong and toxic. *Ayurvedic* physicians generally use mild herbs, because of their nutritive, energetic and therapeutic values. Use of herbs is regarded as the friendly way of treatment, because very less or no side effects are associated with them. That is why it is considered as the most safest and inexpensive healing. Herbs are edible plants in other words concentrated food. Usually they are safe, nutritionally rich and are useful for their content of compounds they can nourish tissues and support the body's own healing process. They are powerful but seldom addictive.

According perfect health is achievable only when body, mind and soul are in harmony with each other and with cosmic surroundings. Since *Ayurveda* is holistic method of healing, it gives ways and means of establishing harmony with society; give more emphasis on one's body constitution and personal health. After knowing all these treatment modalities are designed.

*Ayurveda* is an integral part of Indian culture. Without some awareness of about the theory of *Ayurvedic* medicines and different body purification methods, it is not possible to convince the people about their importance in health.

## Classification of Ayurvedic Herbs

Acharya Charak has given excellent ideal definition of herb and classified Ayurvedic medicines into three groups.

## 1. Food 2. Medicines 3. Poisons

Organic materials useful for the growth i.e. wheat, rice, milk, dates, honey etc. are classified as foods, which are digested and assimilated in body.

Substances, which after entering the body get eliminated from the body via gastrointestinal tract within a specified period of time after their corrective role is over, are termed medicines. This includes most herbs which affect bodily processes, like increased sweating that comes with the use of hot herb ginger, but do not function as foods.

The last group poison is harmful to the tissues and gets absorbed within them, causing many harmful effects. The accumulation of such poisonous substances seriously affects functional capacity of particular body organ and ultimately entire body, which is experienced with various types of heavy metal toxicity in modern polluted environment.

As per Charak Samhita, an ideal herbal medicine should have four qualities.

1. It should be easily available
2. It should have power to eradicate the disease without producing any side effects
3. It should be made into the right direction
4. It should possess all qualities of taste, energy, and post digestive effect to produce desired effect.

It is observed that some food have both nutritional and medicinal properties e.g. barley is a food and also having medicinal value being used as diuretic. Similarly Ashwagandha herb has muscle building property. By this theory all synthetic drugs are poisons and must have side effects, while Ayurvedic medicines being natural of plant origin have no side effect.

Herbs are also classified on the basis of their effect on doshas, dhatus, mala and different systems of the body.

## Properties of Herbs

Like food, all herbs are composed of following three basic factors.

1.  Panchamahabhutas
2.  Six tastes
3.  Twenty attributes

All herbs are grouped into three categories according to their properties, mild, moderate and strong. Strong herbs like bhallataka which causes severe allergic reactions. Herbs with medium potency include herbs with astringent, bitter and pungent taste, like oak bark, cayenne have short term action. On the other mild herbs which include Amla, Brahmi, Ashwagandha etc. can also function as food additives.

## Energy of Herbs

The main energy of herbs is their heating or cooling properties, which is their most powerful and immediate effect upon our bodily functions.

Generally energy follows taste. Pungent, sour and salty tastes are having heating properties, while bitter, astringent and sweet tastes have cooling action.

Heating herbs promote warmth, circulation, digestion, and motivation. In excess they create burning sensation, irritation, seating, thirst, dizziness, fatigue and exhaustion. They increase *pitta(agni)* and decrease *vata* (air) and *kapha*(water).

Cooling herbs create a sense of refreshment. They promote detoxification and clarity. They tend to clear *pitta* and blood but can also increase *vata* and *kapha*. When taken in excess, cooling herbs produce undesirable coldness, sadness, nervousness, poor memory and gradual degeneration. Pungent taste present in chilies, ginger, hot pepper has heating effect. Similarly, yoghurt are also having heating action. Salt is also having heating action.

Sweet taste is cooling as sugar solution counteracts burning sensation in the body. Bitter and cold herbs are often synonymous as bitter herb like gentian reduces fever and inflammation. Astringent taste has constricting, which is the action of something cold like ice. Substances with this taste include alum, bark of oak tree etc. Heating and cooling energy of herbs indicate that these herbs contain energies of fire and water, respectively. Pungent taste is the most heating taste, followed by sour and salty the least. Bitter taste is most cooling, followed by astringent and last is sweet. Generally energy dominates over taste.

## Rasa, Virya Vipica and Prabhava Principle

## Rasa

Rasa means taste of herb. Taste of herb is not incidental, but is an indication of its properties. Different tastes possess different effects. There is general recognition that spicy, pungent herbs tend to be heating or stimulating. Rasa also means 'essence'. Taste thus indicates essence of plant. *Ayurveda* recognizes six main tastes: sweet, sour, salty, pungent, bitter and astringent. These derive from five elements; each taste is composed of two elements. Sweet taste is basically that of sugars and starchs. Sour taste is of fermented or acidic things. Salty is of salts and alkalies. Pungent is the same as spicy or acrid and is often aromatics. Bitter is the bitter herbs like golden seal, gentian. Astringent taste has a constricting quality, as herbs that contain tannin, like oak bark. Any food material or medicine herb put into mouth, the first experience is its taste.

## Virya

Virya is the potency by which the action of a substance takes place. It literally means vigour. Hence any herb devoid of virya will be inactive. It is also seen that often a drug or herb loses its potency after a certain amount of time. This can be owing to the effect of time or improper processing or storage. Virya is the most active attribute of a substance. Out of the twenty primary attributes only eight have the potential to become virya. They are light and heavy, cold and hot, unctuous and rough, and soft and sharp. However, on the basis of concept of agni, virya has ultimately been grouped into two types either cold or hot.

## Vipica

Post digestive effect is inferred from the final action of the ingested food or medicine. The final post digestive effect of taste on body, mind and consciousness is called vipica. Sweet and salty taste have sweet vipica, sour taste has sour vipica, but vipica of pungent, bitter and astringent tastes all are pungent. If one knows the taste, energy and post digestive effect of a herb or food, it is simple to understand its action on bodily systems. This knowledge is essential for healing or cooking. For example, when an individual eats hot chilly pepper, he or she will immediately experience its pungent taste. Heating energy and next day observe the burning sensation in feces and urine.

## Prabhava

Apart from energies, all herbs possess a special healing property, which in called prabhava. It is observed that two types of herbs with same taste, energy, differ in their therapeutic effect; it could be due to action of prabhava. Although it is difficult to explain the exact nature of prabhava Most commonly, it refers to the affinity of an herb for the particular region of the body or for a particular disease. For example tulsi (Basil) is classified as heating herb, but therapeutically helps to clear heat and reduce fever. This means that whatever the cause of fever, tulsi is indicated and this is its prabhava.

## Types of Prabhava

1. Antitoxic: some plants like Shirisha show this type of action.
2. Bactericidal: some plants like guggul, myrrh, garlic have this property.
3. Purgatives: some bitter herbs have this prabhava.

Ghee and milk both are sweet in rasa and vipica and cold in potency, but ghee increases agni, milk does not.

## Dose and Preparation

Ayurvedic herbs can be consumed in any number of ways. The most common way of ingesting them is as powdered dry herb stirred into something mushy and swallowed. The material into which herb is strirred is called vehicle (anupam). The anupam is selected for its ability to pacify the dosha that the medicine is treating and for its ability to carry the herb to the dosha being targeted. The most common vehicles are honey for *kapha*, ghee for *pitta* and warm milk for *vata*. Generally it is advised to take herb alongwith honey to reaxh the herb at target site.

## Therapeutic Effects of Herb

Like allopathic drugs, *Ayurvedic* herbs also have various therapeutic properties like diuretic (increasing in urination), diaphoretic (promoting sweating) etc. All medicinal substances are made up of panchmahabhutas. These substances after entering the body converted into five elements. In elemental state they influence respective dhatus, tissues and systems. The action of these chemical could be localized to any particular organ or systemic affecting the whole body. Also when taken into combined formulae they are more effective. It is rare to find herb sold alone in herbal pharmacies. There are some exceptions like amla, shatawari, ashwangandha etc. Herbs when taken together in formulae viz; virechan churna, sudarshan churna, vatari churna, triphala churna etc. of great therapeutically value.

Selection, dosage of herbal medicine will vary with the patient, which depends upon his/her prakruti, digestive power, age, potency of medicine etc. Herbs are safe and effective, if taken correctly. Rarely some herbs are found unsafe. Long term usage is the key to the herbal medicines, sometimes large dose is required to get the required results. Ghee carries the herb deep into the tissues. Milk counteracts *pitta*. Honey clears cough.

The *Ayurvedic* treatment is entirely based on herbs, which have certain medicinal value or property. In the ancient times, the Indian sages believed that *Ayurvedic* herbs are one-stop solutions to cure a number of health related problems and diseases. They conducted thorough study about the same, experimented with herbs to arrive at accurate conclusions about the efficacy of different plants and herbs that have medical value.

Most of the Ayurvedic herbs, thus formulated are free of side effects or reactions. This is the reason why its popularity grow across the globe. The Ayurvedic herbs that have medicinal quality provide rational means for the treatment of many internal diseases, which are otherwise considered incurable in other systems of medicine. Knowledge of importance of herbs is essential in order to lead a healthy, peaceful and disease-free life.

Therapeutic efficacy of major herbs are summarized in Table 5.1

## Table 5.1 Therapeutic efficacy of Herbs

| 1. For the Brain | 2. For the Heart | 3. For the Respiratory Tract |
|---|---|---|
| Brahmi | Arjuna | Haridra |
| Gotu kola | Guggulu | Vasa |
| Vacha | Kushta | Yashtimadhu |
| Jyotishmati | Pushkaramula | Shirish |
| Sankhapusphi | Hawthrone | |
| 4. For the Stomach | 5. For the liver | 6. For the Urinary Tract |
| Amalaki | Pippali | Punarnava |
| Satawari | Kalamegh | Gokshura |
| Bhringaraja | | Varuna |

| 7. For Genital System(Men) | 8. For Genital System (Female) | 9. For Alimentary Tract |
|---|---|---|
| Ashwagandha | Satavari | Kutaja |
| Kapikacchu | Ashoka | Haritkari |
| | Jipapushpam | *Bibhitaki* |
| | | Bilva |
| **10. Accumulation breaking Herbs** | **11. Tonic Herbs** | **12. Expectorant Herbs** |
| Bheda | Bala | Clove, |
| Kutaj | Aloe | Wild cherry |
| | Kutaj | Eucaluptus |
| | Guduchi | Cardamomom |
| | Golden seal | |
| | Barberry | |
| **13. Disinfectant Herbs** | **14. Antispasmodic, Analgesic Herbs** | **15. Digestive Herbs** |
| Arka | Fennel | Dry ginger |
| Guduchi | Dill | Long pepper |
| Katuka | Papper | Black pepper |
| | Cardamom | Cinnamon |
| | Asafoetida | Chitrak |
| | | Cardamom |
| **16. Antibiotic Herbs** | **17. Antacids Herbs** | **18. Anti Hicuup Herbs** |
| Turmeric | Marshamallow | Long pepper |
| Ginger | | Haritaki |
| Verivert | | |
| **19. Increase Semen Volume** | **20. Anti-emetic Herbs** | **21. Promotes Sweting Herbs** |
| Ashwagandha | Verivert | Basil |
| Gingo biloba | Cardamom | Cinnamon |
| Satavari | Fresh ginger | Ginger |

## Use of Metals in *Ayurveda*

Since ancient times metals are routinely used to treat various diseases. In *Ayurveda* apart from gold other metals that are extensively used which includes silver, arsenic, copper, iron, and zinc. All these metals contain tremendous healing energy. As far as *Ayurveda* is concerned, metals have been used as bhasma (ash). Bhasma literally means anything inorganic or organic burnt into its ash. The process of burning in Ayurvedic terminology is known as calcination. The process of calcination is also employed for preparation of bhasms of coral, shell, pearl. They are oxides or sulphides that are chemically nonreactive to the tissues. Important bhasma includes abhrak, mandur, naga, pravala, rajat, mukta, tambra, vanga, and gold bhasma. *Ayurveda* does not use heavy metals or minerals without extensive processing to render them fit for human consumption. Pure metals contain certain impurities that are toxic to the vital organs such as kidney, liver, spleen and heart. If care is not taken then our vital organs are demaged. That is why purification of metal is very essential. The procedure for the preparation of bhasma is complicated and requires skill, knowledge and experience. All metal and mineral drugs should be purified and rendered safe for the use before being used as drugs. An important bhasma is prepared from mercury, which undergoes 18 stage detoxification and purification processs. *Ayurveda* maintained that bhasma are quickly absorbed in the blood and increase red blood cells. Metals are treated or heated with oil, cow's urine, ghee, butter milk, These ancient methods achieve subtler purification than mere chemical treatments and permit the human tissues to receive the metals without any toxic effects. All major pharmaceutical manufacturers including Dabur, Zandu, Divya Pharmacy, Himalaya, Charak, Baidyanath etc make swarna and other bhasma. Bhasma are catalysts which spark a healing process, hence prescribed in very small doses. Gold is effective nervine tonic. It improves memory and intelligence. Gold bhasma is used in the treatment of diseases such as anaemia, epilepsy, hysteria, heart attack, tuberculosis, leucoderma, loss of memory, rheumatoid arthritis, asthma, etc. Iron is beneficial bone marrow, red blood cells, spleen and liver. Silver promotes strength and stamina. Tin ash is used in diabetes, gonorrhea, syphyilis, asthma, skin diseases, and lung diseases. The efficiency of many herbs increase thousand times when used in conjunction with mercury and sulphur.

# PART II

# SINGLE HERB RASAYANA

# CHAPTER 6

## Amalaki: A Wonder Fruit

---

*Ayurveda* **takes care of the patient as a whole with its holistic approach. Various Ayurvedic herbal and herbomineral preparations are used for the treatment of chronic and degenerative diseases without any side-effect.**

A*mla (Aonla)* is one of the oldest Indian fruits. It is known as Amalaki in Sanskrit. It is a rich source of ascorbic acid (vitamin C). *Vitamin C* found in amla fruits is heat stable, because it is bound to tannins which allow it to be cooked in preparations like chyawanprash a rejuvenating herbal preparation. The fruits of amla have been used in *Ayurveda* as potent Rasayana. Perhaps there is no medicinal plant in nature with such a vast range of medical benefits. It is used as an anti-oxidizing, anti-bacterial and anti-inflammatory agent. Anti-oxidizing property resides in tannoids. It is one of the three constituents of the famous Ayurvedic preparation, *Triphala*, which is prescribed in many digestive disorders. The medicinal properties of *amla* have been elaborately described in ancient Ayurvedic texts, such Charak Samhita and Sushrut Samhita. It is used in making pickles and preserves. Preservation of amla is one of the speciality of the Indian fruit-preservation industry. It is said to be the native of tropical South-Eastern Asia, particularly central and southern India.

# Amla Herb Information

## 1. Nomenclature

Family Name: *Phyllanthaceae*
Scientific Name: *Emblica officinalis* Linn
Sanskit Name: Dhatri, Amalaki
English Name: Indian gooseberry
Common Name: Amalaka, Amrtaphala, Dhatriphala
Synonym: *Phyllanthus emblica*

## 2. Bioenergetics

Rasa: Madhura, Amla, Katu, Tikta, Kasaya
Guna: Laghu, Ruksa
Virya: Shita
Vipaka: Madhura
Karma: Tridosajit, Vrsya, Rasayana, Caksusya

## 3. Biomedical Action

Stimulant, Anti-diabetes, anti-bacterial, anti-viral, Anti-ascorbutic, carminative and stomachic, anti-inflammatory, anti-pyretic, Bactericidal.

## Plant Part Used

Fruits

## Habitat

In Himachal Pradesh, the amla seedlings grow wild in the forests up to elevations of 1,500 m. It is found in dry deciduous forests of India and Burma, and in the extreme north-west, ascending to 1,450 m. It is also found in China and Sri lanka. The major difference between these wild trees and the large-fruited types cultivated in the plains is of winter-hardiness; whereas the improved types are highly susceptible to frost injury, the wild amla are not damaged at all. Amla is a heavy bearer and the fruits also remain free from the attack of birds and wild animals. This plant also remains free from any serious disease and major insect pest.

## Botanical Characters

The Indian gooseberry tree is a small, deciduous tree of small to medium size up to 5.5 m height that has feathery branches. Its bark is usually light brown to black, coming off in thin strips or flakes, exposing the fresh surface of a different colour underneath the older bark; the average girth of the main stem is 70 cm; in most cases the main trunk is divided into 2 to 7 scaffolds very near the base. The berries are fleshy and pale green, and have 6 dimly marked lobes. The flowers appear in dense clusters under the leaves, and hence the fruits grow in the same manner. The tree is indigenous to India. Fruits, fleshy, almost depressed to globose, 2.24 cm in diameter, 5.68 g in weight, 4.92 ml in volume, primrose yellow base.

The stone of the fruit is six ribbed, splitting into three segments, each containing usually two seeds: seeds 4–5 mm long, 2–3 mm wide, each weighing 572 mg, 590 microliters in volume.

## The Flowering and Fruiting Season

The flowering season was observed to occur from the middle of April to the first week of May under Sanwara (H.P.) conditions. The flowering reached its peak in the end of April.

The fruiting season of *amla* is exceptionally long. The fruit in this area become fit for harvesting in December. They can be retained on the tree up to March without any significant loss in quality or yield. The picking of fruits is generally done by the villagers in February and march. In Western India fruiting season is October to December. The average yield of wild *amla*-trees growing in the forests is 23.5 kg. per tree.

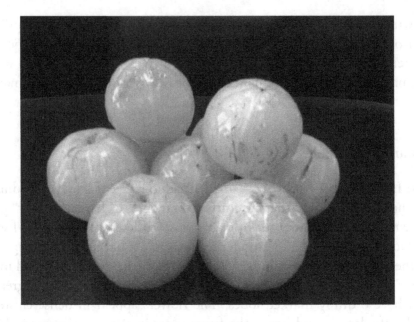

**Amla Fruits**

## Chemical Constituents

A number of laboratory tests conducted on the Indian gooseberry show that for every 100 grams of the berry, it yields between 470 and 680 mg of vitamin C, which increases in case, the juice is extracted. The fruits contains 20 and 15 times more vitamin C than grapefruits and lemon, respectively. Dehydrated berries yield 2.42 to 3.47 g of vitamin C for every 100 g. The fruit, (as well as its bark and leaves) contains a significant amount of tannins too. The seed of the berry contains a fixed oil, essential oil, and phosphatides.

The fruit pulp, which constitutes 90.97 % of the whole fruit, contains 70.5 % moisture. The total soluble solids constitute 23.8 % of the juice. The acidity of *aonla* is 3.28 % on pulp basis. The pulp contains 5.09 % total sugars and 5.08 % reducing sugars. The ascorbic acid content is 1,094.53 mg per 100 ml of juice. The tannins and pectin content of the pulp is 2.73 % and 0.59 %, respectively. The fruit pulp contains 0.75 % protein. The mineral content of the edible portion, as represented by its ash, is 2.922 %. The percentage content of the mineral elements, viz;

phosphorus, potassium, calcium, magnesium, and iron is 0.027, 0.368, 0.059, 0.248 and 0.004, respectively.

## Table 6.1 Analysis of Fruit Pulp of Amla

| Fruit pulp | 90.97% of the whole fruit by weight |
|---|---|
| | 70.5% moisture. |
| Total Soluble Solids (juice) | 23.8% of juice |
| Acidity | 3.28% |
| Total sugars | 5.08% |
| Tannin | 2.73% |
| Pectin | 0.59% |
| Protein | o.75% |
| Minerals (represented by ash) | 2.922% |
| Ascorbic acid | 1094 mg per 100ml of juice |

## Health Benefit

The amla has been an extensive area of research for its medicinal properties. It has been found to prevent and cure the following health disorders.

❖ Amalaki is considered best among Rasayana so called Acharasayana.
❖ It clears all the three doshas present in human body. A regular use of amalaki is presumed to prolong life spans, up to 120 years for humans. Taking one raw amla every day in the morning removes general weakness of different part of the body.
❖ Amla is a rejuvenator for the entire body. The herb is said to stimulate the production of red blood cells, enhance cell rejuvenation, increase lean body mass and support the functions of lever, heart, spleen and lungs.
❖ It has also been used to strengthen eyes, bones and teeth, cause nail and hair to grow.

❖ Amla proves useful in treating various respiratory diseases, especially tuberculosis of the lungs, asthma and bronchitis.

❖ The root bark is useful in ulcerative stomatis. The bark is useful in gonorrhoea, jaundice, diarrhoea and myalgia.

❖ Stimulation of the pancreas, enabling secretion of insulin and consequently reducing blood sugar in diabetes is seen when juice of the berry is taken regularly. So, it is used as a medication for diabetes.

❖ Amla is anti-inflammatory and antipyretic in action.

❖ Amla is a rich source of vitamin C, hense, this amla berry proves to be one of the best medications for scurvy. The powder of dried amla is mixed with an equal quantity of sugar and taken one teaspoon, thrice every day with milk.

❖ The berry is also known to be a preventive measure as well as a balanced remedy for stomach ulcers and tumours.

❖ The leaves are used as infusion with fenugreek seeds in chronic dysentery and as a bitter tonic.

## Other Uses

❖ These fruits are used in huge quantities for making pickles and preserves, both in the villages and in the towns. Several Ayurvedic medicinal preparations, hair wash powders, hair oils etc.

❖ The fruit and bark is also used in tanning of leather by the village tanners. They are offered for sale in the towns for this purpose.

❖ A fixed oil is obtained from the amla is used to strengthen and promote the growth of hair. The dried fruits have a good effect on hair hygiene and have long been used as an ingredient of shampoo and hair oil. Amla is an accepted hair tonic in traditional recipes for enriching hair growth and also pigmentation. The fruit, cut into pieces, is dried, preferably in shade and then boiled in coconut oil, the resulting oil is said to be excellent for preventing hair greying.

❖ An essential oil is distilled from the leaves that are used in perfumery.

❖ The aonla-fruits are dried for making triphala. They are also used as a principal ingredient in making another famous Ayurvedic restorative tonic called Chyawanprash and Brahma Rasayana etc.

❖ The wood is of inferior quality. Used for agricultural implements, poles.

## Home Remedies

❖ The fluid mixture of amla and honey is useful in preserving eyesight. It is valuable in curing conjunctivitis and glaucoma.

❖ One teaspoon of powdered dried amla mixed with 2 teaspoons of jaggery taken twice every day for a month helps treat rheumatism.

❖ A beverage made from the dried fruit, when mixed with lemon juice and misri (sugar candy) eases acute bacillary dysentery.

❖ A decoction of the leaves is used as a chemical-free bactericidal mouthwash. Bark of the root mixed with honey is applied to inflammations of the mouth and a decoction of the leaves is also useful as a mouth wash.

❖ Amla powder is mixed with red sandalwood (*Pterocarpus santalinum)* and prepared in honey to relieve nausea and vomiting.

❖ A paste of the fruit is a useful application to the forehead in cases of headache.

❖ The seed are fried in ghee and ground in conjee (the liquid from boiled rice) is applied to the forehead to stop bleeding from the nose.

❖ The milky juice of the leaves is a good application to sores. Grind the bark of *E. officinalis* (10 g) into a paste and apply to the cut or wound area once daily for 2 to 3 days. Alternatively, squeeze *E. officinalis* leaves and extract the juice to the cut once daily for 3 to 4 days. Healing occurs when the dynamic harmony of the doshas is restored.

❖ To control vomiting mix 2 teaspoonful of amla juice with honey. Take daily.

❖ For treating acidity, a powder consisting of amla, shatavari and sugar in equal parts mixed with equal quantity of honey was prescribed. In adults, the dose of Amalaki powder is 3 to 6 grams.

❖ For the control of gastritis, vomiting, anorexia, take 500 mg to 1 g of amla powder, twice a day to be swallowed on an empty stomach or just before meals with water.

❖ One tablespoon of the paste of amla leaves mixed with honey or buttermilk controls diarrhoea.

❖ A cup of its juice mixed with honey culls intraocular tension extraordinarily. Infusion of the leaves is applied to sore eyes. The dried fruit immersed in water in a new earthen vessel a whole night yields a decoction which is used as a collyrium (a medical lotion applied to the eye as eyewash) in ophthalmia. It may be applied cold or warm.

## Cautions

❖ Amalaki powder is generally a safe medicine. No toxic or adverse effects are reported even with continuous use. It is safe for its use in children and pregnant women. It is also safe to the baby, if the nursing mother is taking this herb powder.

# CHAPTER 7

## *Aloe vera: Ayurveda* Herb with Multiple Benefits

**Ask me what were the secret forces which sustained me during my long fasts. Well, it was my unshakable faith in God, my simple and frugal Lifestyle, and the** *Aloe* **whose benefits I discovered upon my arrival in South Africa at the end of the 19th century.**

Mahatma Gandhi

*Aloe vera* word is originated from Arabic word Aloeh means shining bitter substance and the vera is a Latin word means True, so meaning is True *Aloe*. It is one of the oldest known medicinal plant. The semi-tropical plant, *Aloe vera*, has a long and illustrious history dating back to pre-biblical times. It was originally plant indigenous to South-Central Africa. *Aloe vera* is slimy and mucoid by nature, and cold in action. It is bitter in taste and has a pungent after taste. Therefore in *Ayurveda* it is believed to subside the vitiated *pitta* and *kapha* doshas. The Indian name for *Aloe vera* is kumari (sanskrit) meaning young maiden, which shows its affinity for the female menstrual cycle and its rejuvenative powers for maintaining youthfulness. Some other synonyms as in *Ayurveda* text are Ghritakumari (the fleshly pulp inside the leaves of the herb resembles ghee) and Grihakanya. *Aloe* is a succulent plant widely used in alternative medicine. *Aloe* is big genus which includes at least 420 different plant species. *Aloe vera* specifically refers to the *Aloe barbadensis* Miller plant, which is the most common species used in *Aloe*-based products. Although it is a cactus type plant, it is not cactus. It is a member of liliaceae family. Its closely related member of liliaceae family are onion, garlic, tulip etc. The lower leaf of the plant is used for medicinal purpose. If the lower leaf is sliced open, the gel obtained can be applied on the affected area of the skin. The general public and more and more doctors, therapists and other health professionals all over the world are realizing that *aloe vera* can make a significant and powerful contribution to the improved health and general well-being of millions of people.

## 1. Nomencature

Family – *Liliaceae, Agavaceae*
Scientific Name*: Aloe barbadensis* Mill.
Sanskrit Name: Kumari
English Name: *Aloe vera*, Indian *aloe*
Common Name: Kumarpadhu, Barbados *aloe*, Curacao *aloe*
True *aloe*, West Indian *aloe* etc.

## 2. Bio energies

Rasa: Tikta, Madhura
Guna: Guru, Snigdha,
Virya: Shita
Vipica: Katu

## 3. Biomedical Properties

Anti-inflammatory, antiseptic, antibiotic, anti-microbial, anti-fungal, anti-viral, anti-bacterial, anti-tumor, anti- parasite.

## Habitat

*Aloe vera* has been widely grown as an ornamental plant. The species *aloe vera* is very popular as a medicinal plant with wide spread use both externally and internally against number of diseases. Because of its succulent character, the aloe plant survive in areas of low natural rainfall, making it ideal for low water-use gardens. The species is hardy in nature and can survive almost in dry state, but it can not tolerate very heavy frost or snow. The species exhibits relatively resistant to most insect pests, viz; spider mites, mealy bugs, scale insects, and aphid species may cause a decline in plant health. In pots, the species requires well-drained, sandy potting soil and bright, sunny conditions; however, *Aloe* plants can burn under too much sun or shrivel when the pot does not drain the rain. The use of a good-quality commercial propagation mixture is recommended, as they allow good drainage. Terra cotta pots or earthern pots are preferable as they are porous. In areas that receive frost or snow, the plant is best kept indoors or in heated glasshouses. Large-scale agricultural production of *Aloe vera* is undertaken in India, Australia, Bangladesh, Cuba, the Dominican Republic, China, Mexico, Jamaica, Kenya, Tanzania and South Africa, along with the USA to supply the medicine and cosmetics industry with *Aloe vera* gel.

**Botanical Characters**

*Aloe vera* is a stem less or very short-stemmed succulent plant, grows to a height of 60–100 cm (24–39 in), spreading by offsets. The leaves are thick, fleshy, green to grey-green, with some varieties showing white flecks on their upper and lower stem surfaces. Leaves grow from the base in rosette pattern. Generally each plant has 12 -16 leaves. The plant canbe harvested at an interval of 6 to 8 weeks by removing 3 to 4 leaves per plant. The margin of the leaf is serrated and has small white teeth. The flowers are produced in summer on a spike up to 90 cm (35 in) tall, each flower being pendulous, with a yellow tubular corolla 2–3 cm (0.8–1.2 in) long. Like other *Aloe* species, *Aloe vera* forms arbuscular mycorrhiza which help to draw nutrients and moisture. *Aloe vera* is a succulent plant species that is found only in cultivation, having no naturally occurring wild populations, although closely related *aloe*s do occur in northern Africa. Extracts from *A. vera* are widely used in the cosmetics and alternative medicine industries, being marketed as variously having rejuvenating, healing, or soothing properties.

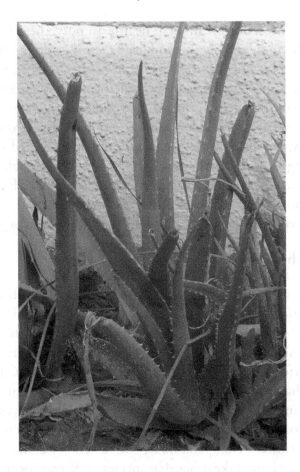

*Aloe vera* **Plant**

## Chemical Constituents

*Aloe vera* leaves contain around 75 phytochemicals such as anthraquinones, enzymes, vitamins, minerals, hormones etc. Anthraquinones are phenolic compounds commonly known for their laxative action. Aloin and emodin both are antraquinines act as analgesics, anti-bacterial and anti-virals. It contains 4 fatty acids. They possess analgesic and antiseptic properties. It also contain auxins and gibberellins hormones that help in wound healing and have anti-inflammatory action. It also provide vitamin A, E, C, which are known antioxidants. It also provides calcium, chromium, copper, selenium, magnesium, manganese, potassium, sodium and zinc. They are essential for the proper functioning of various enzyme systems in different metabolic pathways and few are antioxidants. It provides sugars like glucose, fructose and polysaccharides. *Aloe vera* leaves contains 20 of the 22 amino acids and 7 of the 8 essential amino acids. In addition the plant produces at least six antiseptic agents such as lupeol, salicylic acid, urea nitrogen, cinnamon acid, phenols and sulphur. All of these substances are recognized as antiseptics because they kill or control mold, bacteria, fungi and viruses, explaining why *aloe vera* has the ability to eliminate many internal and external pathogens. That is why these are highly effective in treatment of burns, cuts, scrapes, abrasions, allergic reactions, rheumatoid arthritis, rheumatic fever, acid indigestion, ulcers, plus many inflammatory conditions of the digestive system and other internal organs, including the stomach, small intestine, colon, liver, kidney and pancreas. β-sitosterol is also a powerful anti-cholestromatic which help to lower harmful cholesterol levels, thus helping the heart patients. About 23 polypeptides are present in *Aloe* juice which helps to control a broad spectrum of immune system diseases and disorders. The polypeptides plus the anti-tumour agents, *Aloe* emodin and *Aloe* lectins, are now also used in treatment of cancer.

## Health Benefits

*Aloe* vera has a wide range of benefits.

- ❖ One of the most efficient detoxifying agents
- ❖ A powerful immune system stimulant
- ❖ A strong anti-inflammatory agent
- ❖ An analgesic
- ❖ A stimulator of cell growth
- ❖ An aid to the acceleration tissue healing
- ❖ An antiseptic
- ❖ A rich source of nutrients
- ❖ A powerful aid to the digestive system
- ❖ An Adaptogen

It is the most effective natural plant used both externally and internally and there are numerous benefits that are derived from this wonderful plant.

- ❖ *Aloe vera* because of its blood purification property, it is useful in wounds, edema, pain, inflammation and other skin diseases.
- ❖ It is beneficial in various diseases such as type II diabetes, asthma, jaundice, arthritis, eye disease, tumour, spleen enlargement, liver complaints, vomiting, bronchitis, and ulcers.
- ❖ *Aloe vera* can be used by anyone as it balances all three doshas.
- ❖ *Aloe vera* aids in regulating the menstrual flow in females. Therefore a number of medicines are prepared with *Aloe vera* as the main ingredient since it is sweet, bitter and cooling in action.
- ❖ Three different preparations are made from different part of the plant. The inner gel, the sap and the skin each has its own uses. The inner leaf gel contains 96% water, is anti-inflammatory, antipruritic, vulnerary and hypocholesterolemic. It is drunk as a liquid. A cooling medicine, its soothing nature coats the digestive tract, so it is used to treat ulcers and gastritis. *Aloe* helps clear the toxin out of the digestive system. The cooling nature of the gel reduces acidity. *Aloe* purifies the body and aids liver function, so it is helpful for the skin, when taken internally.
- ❖ *Aloe vera* is also regarded as a Rasayana i.e. that which strengthens the immune system of the body and keeps the disease away.
- ❖ *Aloe* has the ability to penetrate the deepest body tissues (some seven layers deep). This property of *aloe* helps in wound healing.
- ❖ *Aloe vera* aids as natural supportive therapy for maladies of constipation and haemmorrhods. Regular use of *Aloe vera* proves beneficial in both ailments. Kumariasav is a effective natural cure generally prescribed by *Ayurveda* physicians.
- ❖ Relieves constipation, maintains a good gastric pH, helps in inflammatory bowel diseases, non-ulcer dyspepsia, gastric and duodenal ulcers. There are more than 120 drugs made today based on *aloe vera*.
- ❖ Furthermore, the macrophages, monocytes, antibodies and T-cells are stimulated. Phagocytosis (when large white blood cells engulf particles) is dramatically increased to ingest foreign proteins, such as the HIV virus. *Aloe* mucopolysaccharides increase the number and intensity of all immune cells in the body.

❖ It improves joint flexibility and helps in the regeneration of body cells. It strengthens joint muscles, which therefore reduces pain and inflammation in weakened or aged joints

❖ Pharmacologically it is an immunity booster and detoxifies the system. It is recommended in adjuvant therapy with antibiotics, nonsteroidal anti-inflammatory drugs and chemotherapy to eliminate drug induced gastritis and other adverse effects.

❖ It has antiseptic and antibiotic properties which make it highly valuable in treating cuts and abrasions. It has also been commonly used to treat first and second degree burns, as well as sunburns and poison oak, poison ivy, and eczema. It is alleged that sap from *Aloe vera* eases pain and reduces inflammation.

❖ *Aloe vera* gel is useful for dry skin conditions, especially eczema around the eyes and sensitive facial skin.

❖ Its juice may help some people with ulcerative colitis, an inflammatory bowel disease.

❖ *Aloe* has been marketed as a remedy for coughs, wounds, ulcers, gastritis, diabetes, cancer, headaches, immune-system deficiencies, and many other conditions, when taken internally. However, the general internal use is as a laxative. The lower leaf of the plant is used for medicinal purpose. If the lower leaf is sliced open, the gel obtained can be applied on the affected area of the skin.

❖ *Aloe vera* gel has several distinct healing properties. It has the ability to kill certain bacteria, fungi and viruses. It has also the ability to dilate capillaries which increases blood supply in the area to which it is applied. When applied to injured tissues gel penetrates and anaesthetizes tissue relieving pain and itching. *Aloe Vera's* anti-inflammatory properties reduce swelling of the skin and muscles.

❖ *Aloe vera* contains salicylic acid, phenols, sulphur etc. These compounds exhibit inhibitory effect against number of bacteria, fungi and viruses.

❖ *Aloe* gel is used as skin tonic against pimples. It is uised for soothing the skin.

There is wide range of applications and beneficial effects of its use, continue to increase the popularity of ancient plant.

**Other Uses**

❖ It can also be used as a hair styling gel and works especially well for curly or fuzzy hair.

❖ It is also used for making makeup, moisturizers, soap, shampoos and lotions.

**Home Remedies**

❖ The juice extracted from the pulp of the herb can be applied on the skin in case of burns and it provides both soothing as well as healing benefits.

❖ Add *Aloe* leaves to hot water and boil, inhaling steam to relieve chest congestion..

❖ Drink *Aloe* juice to relieve indigestion, heartburn, acid reflux, bloating.

❖ After keeping the pulp of *Aloe vera* in a container for some time, the juice would separate from the same. This may be taken three or four times in a day as an effective home remedy for urine infection., flatulence, peptic ulcers and constipation.

❖ For inflammation in the skin tissue along with pain and swelling, Mix some turmeric powder into the pulp of *Aloe vera* and this has to be heated on fire and can be applied to the affected part for relief.

❖ Apply externally and drink juice to relieve haemorrhoids.

❖ Eliminate UTI and prostate problems by drinking *Aloe vera*.

❖ Consume 1-2 teaspoonful of fresh gel daily for young and healthy skin.

❖ Ayurvedic texts it has been said that the fresh juice applied on the face can result into fairness and loss of blemishes.

# CHAPTER 8

## Ashoka: A Divine Tree

---

"We can't talk about our own health without understanding our place in our environment, because in order to fulfill our potential we have to live in the context of our surroundings. We have to know our place in the ecosystem of which we are a part, and this means living 'consciously': being aware of nature and how it affects us and how we, in turn, affect nature."

Sebastian Pole

Ashoka is a member of divine club along with arjuna, clove and others, used in *Ayurveda*. It's botanical (Latin) name is *Saraca asoca* (Roxb.), De wild. or *Saraca indica* belonging family *Caesalpiniaceae*. It is a purely sattvic herb. Ashoka's flowers are described in sanskrit as hemapushpa (filled with golden, divine light, like the colour of the morning rising sun, or the light of the soul). Ashoka is regarded as highly effective Ayurvedic medicine for number of diseases. As the name suggest Ashoka removes grief from our heart. This is not the physical property, but it is spiritual energy of the herb. The meaning of word Ashoka is no grief "A" means no and "shoka" means grief. So the literal meaning of the word Ashoka is that removes shoka. It is like in presence of light darkness disappears. Similarly in presene of ashoka tree grief does not exhist. Ashoka tree has been mentioned in some of the oldest Indian spiritual literature apart from *Ayurveda*. This tree can be found all over the Indian subcontinent across India, Ashoka tree has been mentioned in some of the oldest Indian literature apart from *Ayurveda*. Ashoka tree is believed to be sacred and apart from Ramayana, Ashoka tree is mentioned in Buddhism and Jainism as well. Charak Samhita which is believed to have been composed in 1000 BC describes about Ashoka tree and its medicinal benefits. In the Ramayana, one of the important book of Hindu mythology, there is mention of Ashoka tree and Gautam Buddha- Indian philosopher and founder of buddhism was said to be born under this tree. in the 6th century B.C. The tree is worshipped by all hindus as well as Buddhists. Because it is a sacred tree, is planted near temple. The tree is symbol of love and is dedicated to Kamdev, the Indian God of love.

## Ashoka Herb Information

## 1. Nomenclature

Family Name: *Caesalpiniaceae*
Scientific Name: *Saraca asoca* (Roxb.), De wild, *Sarcaca indica*
Sanskrit Name: Shoka, Ashoka, Asupala, Anganapriya
English name: Ashoka
Common name: Ashoka, Ashoka Tree, Anganapriya, Asogam, Asokada, Ashopalava, Asok, Asoka, Asoka Tree, Asupala, Gandapushpa, Kankelli, Kenkalimara, Thawgabo, Vichitrah

## 2. Bioenergetics

Rasa: Tikta, Kasaya, Madhura
Guna: Laghu, Ruska
Virya: Shita
Vipaka: Katu
Karma: Hridaya, Vishaghna, Grahi, Varnya, Sothahara
Dosha effect: *Kapha* and *Pitta*
Dhatu: Blood, Muscle, Fat and Reproductive System
Srotas: Circulatory and Reproductive System

## 3. Biomedical Action

Anti-cancer, anti-menorrhagia, anti-oxytoxic, anti–microbial

## Habitat

The Ashoka tree is a rainforest tree. It is found throughout India. It is known to grow at an altitude of 750 m above the sea level. The tree is believed to have originated in the Western ghats and deccan plateau. It can also be found in central and eastern Himalayas. The plant requires medium to deep well drained fertile soils, slightly acidic to neutral soils for good growth. It grows well in tropical to sub-tropical situations under irrigation This is a perennial plant which can range from dark green to greyish green in colour, especially in Himalaya, Kerala, Bengal and whole south region. In Maharashtra it is distributed in Tilari, Sawantwadi, Matheran, Kolhapur, Ramghat. In Himalaya, it is found at Khasi, Garo and Lussi hills and in Kerala region it is found in Patagiri, Kaikatty & Pothundi of Palakkad district, Thrisur, Kollam and Kannaur districts is found wild along streams or in shade of the evergreen forests. Indigenous to India, Sri-lanka, Burma and Malaysia. Earlier it was distributed throughout India up to an altitude of 720 m., but now it is left wild in sporadic patches.

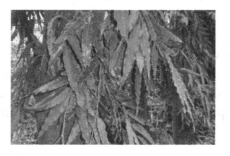

**Ashoka Tree**

## Botanical Characters

Ashoka is slow-growing, small, evergreen, erect tree 6 - 10 m high. Leaves are narrowly lanceolate 15 to 25 cm. long ; cork like at the base and with a short petiole. Bark is smooth grey-brown or almost black. The bark of *Saraca indica* is distinguished by presence of warty protuberances on its outer surface. Flowers are fragrant. The crown is compact and shapely. The Ashoka flowers from February to April. The flowers appear in lush and heavy bunches The plant is prized for its beautiful foliage and flowers. The flowers are bright golden to pink-red in colour with a diameter of 7 to 10 cm and they turn before wilting. Red stamens come out of the flower, 7 to 8. Flowering occurs in Spring season and Fruition occurs in early winter. The pods are 10 to 25 cm long, 3.7 to 5 cm wide and flat. There are 4 to 8 flat seeds, 3.7 cm long. This tree has an important role in Indian cultural traditions.

## Chemical Constituents

The stem bark is chiefly used in medicines and it has been reported to contain chemicals such as glycoside, flavonoids, tannins, saponins, alkanes, esters and primary alcohols. The alcoholic extracts present in the bark have shown a significant action against wide range of bacteria. The Ashoka tree's dried bark contains tannins, sterol, catechol, and other organic calcium compounds. The powered bark of the tree also contains aluminum, strontium, calcium, iron, magnesium, phosphate, potassium, sodium, and silica. Recent analysis of the dry powdered bark showed the presence of a fair amount of tannin and probably an organic substance containing iron. No active principles of the nature of alkaloid, essential oil, etc., were found. Bark contains a fair amount of tannin and catachin. In order to maintain the medicinal values and physicochemical properties of the Ashoka herb, it is suggested that they be kept in air tight containers, protected from light, moisture, and contamination from microbes.

## Plant Part Used

Flower and stems dried and bark dried and fresh Use

## Health Benefits

Ashoka or *Saraca indica*, has many health benefits and has long been used in traditional Indian medicine as a key ingredient in various therapies and cures. Various studies on extracts from Ashoka bark provide evidence of its several health benefits.

❖ It can fight fever, cold and infections as it possesses anti-bacterial properties.

❖ *Ayurveda* has been using Ashoka for menorrhagia traditionally. A preparation made from Ashoka tree known as Ashokarishta is given for this disease and also for uterine infections. It helps stop vaginal bleeding. The Ashoka herb benefits the endometrium and uterine muscles and this makes it effective as a uterine tonic for irregular menstrual cycles and miscarriage.

❖ The methanol extracts from Ashoka showed positive results against rheumatic arthirits. Ashoka bark has been traditionally used as a remedy for internal hemorrhoids.

❖ It is also effectively used in *Ayurveda* for clearing congestion from the medas dhatus and mamsa, especially when there may be leucorrhoea, endometriosis, cysts, and fibroids from excess *kapha* and *ama* in the menstrual disorder.

❖ Specific analgesic properties present in Ashoka can be used to calm the nerves when they have been aggravated by the *vata*.

❖ *Ashoka* herb is also said to improve the complexion of skin. This herb can be used to obtain relief from burning sensations on the skin. It also helps to get rid of the toxins from the body.

❖ Natural pain relief through increasing oxygen and circulation to painful areas. Applications for lower back, knee, elbow, neck and shoulders.

❖ Dried flowers of Ashoka are used for diabetes treatment. The bark of the tree is used to treat scorpion bite.

❖ The leaves and bark are used to get rid of worms in stomach. Leaves possess blood purifying properties. Flowers used in dysentery and diabetes.

❖ Keeps your breath fresh and taste sharp for better digestion.

## Home Remedies

❖ An extract of the Ashoka flower can be made by grinding the flowers along with some water. Doses of 15–60 drops can be taken. This is a effective remedy to treat haemorrhagic dysentery.

❖ Decoction of the bark is prepared by boiling 113 g of the bark in 113 ml of milk and 434 ml of water till the water is evaporated.

Take this with milk in two or three divided doses during the
course of the day in menorrhagia. Start it from the 4th day of the
monthly period. Continue taking this till the bleeding ceases. in
purifying the blood naturally and in preventing skin allergies.

# CHAPTER 9

## Ashwagandha: A Magical Adaptogenic Herb

All plants contain adaptogenic/tonic compounds. Because plants have to contend with a good deal of stress themselves.

James Duke

Ashwagandha also known as *Withania somnifera* Dunal. Ashwgandha is a sanskrit word, ashwa means horse; gandha means fragrance. It indicates the the strength and sexual vitality of the horse. It is popularly known as Indian ginseng, or winter cherry has been used for centuries in *Ayurveda*. Charak has classified ashwagandha as Rasayana. It increases youthfulness, longevity and vitality It is a reputed health food and herbal tonic and used for cardiovascular diseases. Ashwagandha is used either as a single herb or one of the ingredient of polyherbal or herbomineral formulations. In the current decade, there has been an extensive research on its effect against number of diseases. Ashwagandha herb has been used as an aphrodisiac, liver tonic, anti-inflammatory agent, astringent, and more recently to treat bronchitis, asthma, ulcers, emaciation and insomnia. Ashwagandha is used in *Ayurveda* medicine as a rejuvenative herb, used in conditions of weakness to strengthen the body. Ashwagandha has a traditional reputation as a tonic or adaptogenic herb with multiple, nonspecific actions that counteract the effects of stress and generally promote wellness. It is used in formulation to provide vital energy while other herbs and minerals take effect. Compound known as glcowithanolides and alkaloids are believed to account for its medical applications.

## Ashwagandha Herb Information

### 1. Nomenclature

Family Name: *Solanaceae*
Botanical Name: *Withania somnifera Dunal*
Sanskrit Name: Ashwagandha
English Name: Winter cherry
Common Name: Winter cherry, Ashwagandha, Withania, Indian Ginseng, Ashgand, Achuvagandi Ashgandh, Ajagandha, Kanaje

### 2. Bioenergies

Rasa: Tikta, Kasaya, Madhura
Guna: Laghu, Ruska
Virya: Usna
Vipica: Madhu
Karma: Hridaya, Vishaghna, Grahi, Varnya, Sothahara
Dosha effect: KV +
Dhatu: Blood, Muscle, Fat, Bone and Reproductive System
Srotas: Reproductive, Nervous, Respiratory

### 3 Biomedical Action

Tonic, nervine, sedative, nerve restorative, adaptogen, aphrodisiac, anti-inflammatory, antioxidant, immunomodulation, free radical scavenger, anti-stress, rejuvenative, hypotensive, anti-spasmodic, anti-arthritic.

### Habitat

It is found in dry areas of India and Africa. The plant is grown in various places of India. It is also cultivated in Pakistan, Bangladesh, Nepal and Sri Lanka; parts of India like Madhya Pradesh, Rajasthan, Punjab, Haryana, Uttar Pradesh, Gujarat and Maharashtra.

## Botanical Characters

Ashwagandha is a small, erect woody branched shrub in the Solanaceae family. It grows about 1.25 m in height; thickness vary with age. Ashwagandha stem is terate, branched, cylindrical, solid; roots are straight, unbranched, thickness varying with age. Stem bases variously thickened. The roots when dry are cylindrical, gradually tapering down with a brownish white surface and pure white inside when broken. The roots are the main portion of the plant used therapeutically. The leaves are simple, petiolate, ovate, acute, entire and up to 10 cm. Ashwagandha flowers are complete, hermaphrodite, 4- 6 mm in diameter, lucid-yellow or greenish. Its flowering time is in winter. Ashwagandha fruit is a berry enclosed in the green persistent calyx, 5 mm in diameter, smooth, more or less globose, green when unripe, orange-red coloured in ripening stage. The bright red fruit is harvested in the late fall and seeds are dried for planting in the following spring.

## Chemical Constituents

Roots are the principal parts which are used therapeutically, scientists have studied detailed chemistry and vide variety of chemical constituents have been reported. The biologically active chemical constituents are alkaloids, (isopelletierine, anaferine), steroidal lactones (withanolides, withaferins), saponins and withanolides. At present, 35 withanolides, 12 alkaloids and several sitoindosides from ashwagandha plant have been isolated and studied. Important constituents includes somniferine, somnine, somniferinine, withananine, anhydrine, withanolides, methanol, hexane, diethyl ether, alkaloid (0.13-0.31%), choline, tropanol, pseudotopanol, cuscokygrene, 3-tigioyloxytropana, isopelletierine, withaferin-A, starch, glycosides, dulcitol, withancil, aspartic acid, glycine, tyrosine, alanine, glutamic acid, cysteine. Withanolides are believed to be active principle which account for the multiple medicinal application of Ashwagandha. It stimulates the activation of immune system cells such a lymphocytes. It inhibits inflammation and improves memory. Taken together, these actions support the traditional reputation of Ashwagandha as a tonic or adaptogens.

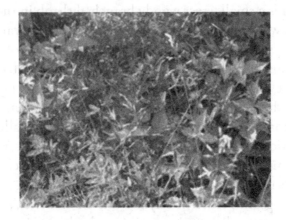

**Ashwagandha Plant**

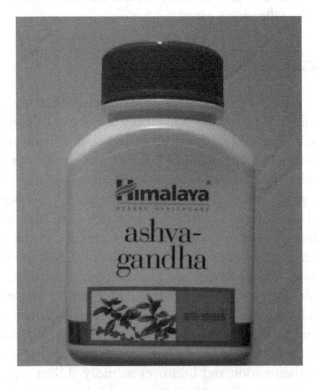

**Ashwagandha Product**

## Plant Part Used: Roots

Traditionally all parts of the plant are used as herbal remedies but the root, which has a damp horse smell, is much more effective.

## Health Benefit

Ashwagandha a popular medicinal herb is widely used for health, vitality, longevity, and rejuvenation purpose.

- ❖ In one clinical trial significant improvement was observed in red blood cell count, haemoglobin, hair melanin and seated stature with daily dose of 3 g. of ashwagandha powder in healthy males. Daily intake of herb reduced serum cholesterol and maintained calcium level; ESR was decreased significantly with improvement in sexual performance.
- ❖ In one laboratory study anxiolytic and anti-depressant action of ashwagandha was compared with lorazepam and imipramine standard pharmaceutical drugs. Both ashwagandha and lorezapam reduced level of anxiety. Ashwagandha also shown reduction in depression.
- ❖ A decrease in blood glucose comparable with hypoglycemic drug was noticed with ashwagandha roots with type II diabetes patients. Significant increases in urine sodium, urine volume, and decreases in serum cholesterol, triglycerides, and low-density lipoproteins were also seen.
- ❖ A laboratory study with laboratory animals revealed ashwagandha has a thyrotropic effect
- ❖ Roots of ashwagandha exhibited improvement in auto-immune conditions, rheumatoid arthritis, and osteo arthritis, cancer, and chronic connective tissue disorders.
- ❖ Ashwagandha appears to possess both immunosuppressive and immunotonic abilities and is therefore it is called a 'true' adaptogens.
- ❖ It is an anabolic muscle builder. As it benefits all muscle tissues, it is used as a heart tonic, uterine tonic, lung tonic as well as

for increasing muscle weight and tone in convalescents, slow developing children and the elderly people.

❖ Withania possess a powerful anti-stressor effect and provide cardioprotection similar to ginseng a known adaptogen. It also increases heart weight and level of glycogen in liver. It has a specific affinity for the majja dhatu. It is beneficial in stress related disorders, like arthritis, hypertension, diabetes, general debility.

❖ Because of presence of large amount of lipids in brain and nervous system, they are relatively more vulnerable to free radical damage. Brain uses nearly 20% of the total oxygen supply. Free radical damage of nervous tissue may contribute to neuronal loss in cerebral ischemia and may be involved in normal aging and neurodegenerative diseases, It works as Rasayana that helps in preventing early aging and rejuvenates the whole body.

❖ Recent studies revealed that ashwagandha root contains steroidal properties which can be effective in treating inflammation. It is also used to treat low back pain and sciatica.

❖ Withania is helpful in relieving insomnia and possess mild sedative properties that help to promote sound sleep.

❖ It is highly effective in healing wounds and injuries.

❖ Because of its good penetrating powers, ashwagandha herb promotes mental calmness and satisfaction.

❖ Since the herb is a powerful aphrodisiac, it assists in enhancing sexual powers and promotes long-lasting endurance. It helps in increasing the number and quality of sperms.

❖ It revitalizes the body and decreases untimely fatigue that is caused due to weak body strength, which results from accumulation of negative energies in the body.

❖ Due to presence of *vata*-suppressant properties, Ashwagandha relieves stress and helps in nurturing nervous system.

❖ The roots of *W. somnifera* are alterative, aphrodisiac, deobstruent, diuretic, narcotic, sedative and restorative in nature.

❖ *Withania* provides nourishment to the brain for better functioning and greater ability to work.

❖ It helps in improving mental ability and mental concentration, gaining retaining power and increasing the production of bone marrow.

❖ It also helps to reduce a bad cholesterol level which is responsible for hypertension and cardiovascular problems.

❖ It is used as a liver tonic and anti-inflammatory agent that treats asthma, ulcers, insomnia.

❖ According to one research report, incorporation of the herb in the diet prevents or decreases the growth of tumours in humans.

❖ In one laboratory trial on rats, it was found that ashwagandha favourably alters blood and urine glucose levels, haemoglobin and liver enzymes in diabetic rats

❖ In clinical study evaluating the effect of ashwagandha on the processs of aging on 50-59 years olds for period of one year was significantly slowed down in number of parameters.

❖ Ashwagandha roots powder can be an effective herbal supplement for the treatment of cancer. It has the ability to slow tumour growth.

❖ An ointment prepared by boiling the leaves in fat is useful for bedsores and wounds. Leaves have been reported to be anti-inflammatory agent. In addition to its medicinal use, Ashwagandha is also extensively used at home in the form of tea.

## Ayurvedic Approach

1. According to Ayurvedic system there are saptadhatu (seven tissues) manufactured by body namely lymph, blood, bone, muscle, fat, nerve and reproductive tissues. Within thirty days, through series of enzymatic processes lymph is transformed into ojas(life essence), which is the body's most specialized tissue. Ojas controls immunity, reproduction, and general health and ashwagandha specially builds ojas and supports these functions.

2. One of the special properties of ashwagandha is that it will boost ojas. Ojas is the most subtle, refined level of the physical body and is the end result of properly digested healthy food. It is a by-product of healthy, efficient, contented physiology. Ojas is the essence of seven dhatu or body tissues. It is responsible for a

healthy immune system, physical strength, lustrous complexion, clarity of mind and sense of Well-being. It allows consciousness to flow within the body. With decreased ojas, we are less in touch with ourselves and more prone to diseases and having a feeling of disharmony.

3.  Ojas improves aging parameter such as graying hair, calcium level and increased libido & sexual function; prevents stress related gastrointestinal ulcers, increases physical endurance and prevents the depletion of vitamin C and cortisol. Ojas depletion can be caused by stress, which triggers stress fighting hormones and free radicals that in turn cause degeneration of the immune and other physiological systems. This stress induced reaction can open the gate way for illness and disease.

4.  It is helpful with fatigue and nervous exhaustion and increases digestive heat in chronic conditions. Ashwagandha is the herb of choice in arthritis, which involves joints that are painful, dry, swollen and inflamed,

5.  Ashwagandha is effective for insomnia but does not act as a sedative. Its rejuvenative and nervine properties produce energy which in turn help the body to settle and sleep. Thus it helps the body to address a stress related condition rather than masking it with sedatives. A herb that rejuvenates the nervous system, erases insomnia and eases stress.

6.  It has been found that Ashwagandha increases the number of immune cells known as T cells and B cells helping to fight infections. All these actions directly oppose the effects of stress. It increases red blood cell counts, improves hemoglobin level, increases endurance and stamina and increases lean body weight.

7.  Many people have compared ashwagandha with Chinese ginseng, but modern science studies have shown ashwagandha to be superior to ginseng.

## Home Remedies

❖ A fomentation of the leaves is used for sore eyes, boils, and swollen hands and feet.

❖ Paste of the leaves is locally applied to kill lice infesting the body, and over carbuncles (An acute suppurative inflammation of the skin and tissues under the skin, rapidly spreading around the original point of infection) and syphilitic sores.

## Cautions

❖ Do not take Ashwagandha, if you are suffering from congestion.
❖ In case you are pregnant or breast-feeding, do not use the herb.

# CHAPTER 10

## Bala: A Cure for Parkinson's Disease

---

One of the biggest tragedies of human civilization is the precedents of chemical therapy over nutrition. It's a substitution of artificial therapy over nature, of poisons over food, in which we are feeding people poisons trying to correct the reactions of starvation.

Royal lee

Bala or *Sida cordifolia Linn* is an important plant in *Ayurveda* system of medicine. Bala is a Sanskrit word which means strength. It is also known as an Aphrodisiac. The species name, cordifolia, refers to the heart-shaped leaf. It is used for weight loss, and boosting physical endurance and strength. It is often used by athletes and bodybuilders. This is a sweet, cold and heavy herb that builds immunity. Bala contains five out of the six tastes, a rare property, so it is widely used to nourish all body tissues (sapta dhatus). Bala is soothing and mucilaginous, so particularly used against *vata* nerve disorders and it is combined with other tonics for specific organs such as with arjuna for heart.

**Bala Herbal Information**

**1. Nomenclature**
Family Name: *Malvaceae*
Scientific Name: *Sida cordifolia*
Sanskrit Name: Bala
English name: Country Mallow

Common name: Kungyi, bala, country mallow, heart-leaf sida, flannel weed.

## 2. Bio-energetics

Rasa: Madhura
Guna: Laghu, snigdha, picchila
Viyra: Shita
Vipaka: Madhura
Dosha: VPK=

Karma: Vata*pitta* shamak, Vedanasthapana, Shotahara, Balya, Vatahara, Grahi, Hrudya, Raktapitta shamak, shukrala, Prajasthapana, Mutrala, Jvaragna, Balya, Brumhana, Ojovardhak

## 3. Biomedical Action

Diaphoretic, diuretic, anti-asthmatic, stimulating, strengthening, energizing, anti-pyretic, anti-ulcer, anti-inflammatory.

## Habitat

It is a weed of roadsides and wasteland found in all districts. Bala is a perennial subshrub of the mallow family *Malvaceae* native to India. It is distributed throughout tropical and sun tropical India and Sri lanka, growing wild along the roadside in villages. It has naturalized throughout the world, and is considered an invasive weed by invasive groups in Africa, Australia, the southern United States, Hawaiian Islands, New Guinea, and French Polynesia. Since it is unwanted weed, it competes with the cultivated crop for nutrients, light, humidity.

## Botanical Characters

*S. cordifolia* is an erect perennial plant grows to about 0.5 to 2.0m (20 to 79 in) in length. The entire plant covered with soft white felt-like hair that is responsible for one of its common names, "flannel weed",

The stems are yellow-green, hairy, long and slender. The yellow-green leaves are oblong covered with hairs, and 3.5 to 7.5 cm (1.4 to 3.0 in) long by 2.5 to 6 cm (0.98 to 2.4 in) wide. The flowers are dark yellow, sometimes with a darker orange center. As a weed, it invades cultivated fields, competing with main cultivated crop. The roots of Sida are 5 to 13 cm long and about 0.62 cm in diameter.

## Plant Parts Used

Roots, fruits, leaves and seeds

## Chemical Constituents

S. cordifolia whole plant contains alkaloids to the extent of 0.085 %. A study reported 0.112% of alkaloid in whole plant. Seeds contain much higher quantities i.e.,0.32 % of alkaloid, than either the stems, leaves or roots. The principal portion of alkaloid was identified to be ephedrine. The seeds contain 3.23% fatty oils, seed oil contains sterculic, malvalic and coronaric acids.

## Health Benefits

Bala has numerous health benefits

- ❖ Bala plant extract exhibited significant improvement in functioning of heart by stabilizing the heart rhythm.
- ❖ In *Ayurveda* bala herb is used as medicine for asthmatic bronchitis, nasal congestion, and inflammation of oral mucosa. Plant extract of bala when administered, it significantly reduced inflammation and pain.
- ❖ Aqueous extract of the herb stimulates regeneration of lever in mice.
- ❖ Bala has antipyretic and anti-ulcerogenic properties.
- ❖ Ethanoic extract of bala exhibited potent antioxidant and anti-inflammatory activity.

❖ The roots, seeds and leaves all are used in medicine. Roots are regarded as cooling, astringent, stomachic and tonic. Seeds are considered aphrodisiac and are used in gonorrhoea, cystitis, and also given for colic. The leaves are used for ophthalmia. The juice of the whole plant is used in rheumetism.

❖ In India, this plant has been used for a very long time to cure diseases such as bronchial asthma, cold and flu, chills, headache, nasal congestion, aching joints and bones, wheezing.

❖ Laboratory studies were undertaken to study the efficacy of bala plant extracts in controlling diabetes. Results demonstrate significant lowering of blood sugar after administration of the extracts of bala plant. The results also indicate possible weight loss as fat cells loose fat.

❖ The juice obtained from the roots is applied to unhealthy sores. Decoction of the roots bark is given in sciatica and rheumatism. The paste of its leaves is applied in ophthalmic diseases. It is also rejuvenative, nutritive and stimulant to the heart.

❖ Parkinson's disease is a brain disorder which is characterized by severe shaking of the body. This is a neurological disorder. *Ayurveda* prescribes treatments for this which include diet, massage therapy and medical formulations. Bala is one of the herbs which are used in medicinal formulations for Parkinson's disease and controlling Parkinson at appreciable level.

❖ It is diuretic, diaphoretic, anti-asthmatic, stimulating to the central nervous system.

❖ The stem of the plant generally contains essential oils and 1-2 % alkaloids composed mainly of stimulants, which are known to be excellent for weight loss.

❖ It lowers the blood pressure and improves cardiac irregularity. It is used in the popular medicine for the treatment of stomatitis of asthma and nasal congestion

❖ Bala is sweet in taste and hot in action. It nourishes and strengthens immunity, heals the nerves, reduces pain and stimulates formation of healthy new tissue.

❖ Leaves are cooked and eaten in case of bleeding piles.

## Cautions

❖ Ayurvedic formulations containing *S.cordifolia* should not be prescribed with cardiac glycosides, monoamine oxidase inhibitors but owing to variation of active constituent, great care should be taken while prescribing *S.cordifolia* with cardiac glycosides.

# CHAPTER 11

## Basil: A Holy Plant

---

"Listen to your being. It is continuously giving you hints; it is a still, small voice. It does not shout at you, that is true. And if you are a little silent you will start feeling your way. Be the person you are. Never try to be another, and you will become mature. Maturity is accepting the responsibility of being oneself, whatsoever the cost. Risking all to be oneself, that's what maturity is all about."

Osho

Basil is a member of the *Ocimum* genus, The genus name, *Ocimum*, derives from the ancient Greek word, okimon, meaning smell which suggests the uniqueness of basil's fragrance. Because of its unique flavour the name basil is coined, which is originated from the Greek word Basileus which means king so the literal meaning is king of royal fragrance. The basil var. *Ocimum tunaiflorum* previously known as *Ocimum sanctum* is a sacred herb in Hindu philosophy. Basil is fairly large genus includes 60 annual species. Basil is rarely used in Indian cuisine, but it is very important feature to Vietnamese, Thai Italian, Cambodian, Taiwan and Laotian cultures. In Hindu houses, basil is the protecting spirit of the family. Every religious Hindu go to rest, a tulsi leaf is placed in his mouth. For Hindu, the British at one time, used tulsi as a substitute for a Bible for taking oath in a court of law. In Malaysia basil is planted on the grave. All *Ocimum* species yield essential oils which is responsible for the medicinal uses including antimicrobial, antioxidant, antifungal and anti-inflammatory activities. Modern research has classified tulsi as an adaptogenic herb which have been shown to support the body's natural immune system.

## Basil Herb Information

### 1. Nomencalture

Family Name: *Lamiaceae* (mints)
Scientific Name: *Ocimum basilicum, Ocimum tenuiflorum*
Sanskrit Name: Tulsi
English Name: Basil, Saint Joseph's Wort
Common Name: Tulsi, Basil, Thai Basil, or Sweet Basil

### 2. Bioenergies

Rasa: Katu
Guna: Laghu, Tikshna, Ruksha
Virya: Usna
Vipica: Katu
Dosha effect: VK -, P +
Dhatu (tissue): Plasma, Blood, Reproductive, Bone marrow

### 3. Biomedical Action

Anti-inflammatory, anti-bacterial, analgesic, anti-depressant, anti-spasmodic, anti-venomous, carminative, cephalic, diaphoretic, digestive, emmenagogue, expectorant, febrifuge, insecticide, nervine, stomachic, sudorific, tonic and stimulant.

### Habitat

Basil is originally native to India, it is believed to be in cultivation for more than 5,000 years. It is a half-hardy annual plant, best known as a culinary herb. Basil grows wild as a perennial on some pacific islands otherwise it is annual. It is believed that in the sixteenth century Basil was brought from India to Europe through the Middle East. Subsequently to America in the seventeenth century. There are many varieties of *O. basilicum*, as well as several related species or hybrids also called basil.

The basil comes in many different varieties, each with its own unique botanical characters and unique flavour. Because of distinct flavour, basil is mainly used in culinary. In the Italian food typically sweet basil is used. While in Thailand basil (*O. basilicum* var. thyrsiflora) is used. Other varities of basil are lemon basil (*O.basillium* var citriodorum) and holy basil (*O. tenuiflorum*), which are used in Asia. While most of common varieties of basil are annuals, some are perennial in warm, tropical climates, including holy basil.

**Botanical Characters**

There is wide variation between varieties within the genus. Basil attain a height between 30-130 cm. The leaves are 3-11 cm long and 1 -6 cm broad, opposite, edge of the leaf blade has teeth, yellowish green to dark green in colour, silky in texture. The flowers are small white to purple in colour. They are arranged at the end of branches. The fruits are dry but does not split open when ripe.

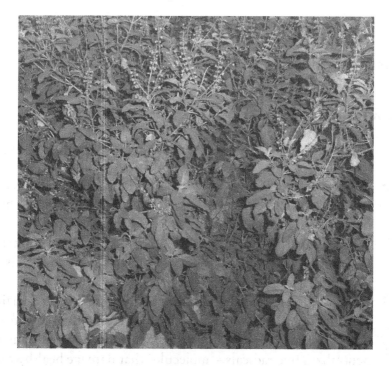

**Basil Plant**

**Chemical Constituents**

Basil leaves contain essential oils such as eugenol, limonene, citronellol, linalool, citral, and terpineol with several health benefits. These compounds are known to have anti-inflammatory and anti-bacterial properties. Basil herb contains remarkably high levels of beta-carotene, vitamin A, cryptoxanthin, lutein and zea-xanthin. These compounds are very very powerful antioxidants, they act as protective scavengers against oxygen-derived free radicals and reactive oxygen species (ROS) that play a role in aging and various disease processes. Zeaxanthin is a powerful yellow flavonoid compound, that protects the eye by absorbing damaging blue light and reducing glare. It is known that blue light can cause harmful oxidative stress in the eye. Zeaxanthin protects cells and membranes by reducing harmful free radicals. Studies suggest that common herbs, fruits, and vegetables that are rich in zea-xanthin anti-oxidant help to protect from age-related mascular disease (AMRD), especially in the elderly persons.

**Plant Parts Used**

Leaves, roots and seeds are seldom used.

**Health Benefits**

Since ancient times basil is extensively used against number of diseases.

❖ Basil leaves contain many notable plants derived chemical compounds that are known to have disease preventing and health promoting properties.
❖ The herb's parts are very low in calories and contain no cholesterol, but are very rich source of many essential nutrients, minerals, and vitamins that are required for optimum health.
❖ One hundred gram (100g) of fresh basil leaves contain amazingly 5.275 g vitamin A which is 175 % of daily adult requirement of vitamin A. Beta carotene is a powerful antioxidant that neutralizes free radicals – molecules that damage healthy cells – and increases the risk of accelerating the aging process and/or

health conditions. It promotes the growth of strong teeth and bone, is essential for the formation of visual purple, a pigment that allows you to see in dim light.

❖ Vitamin K in basil is essential for many coagulant factors in the blood and plays a vital role in the bone strengthening function by helping mineralization process in the bones.

❖ Basil herb contains a good amount of minerals like potassium, manganese, copper, and magnesium. Potassium is an important component of cell and body fluids, which helps control heart rate and blood pressure. Manganese is used by the body as a co-factor for the antioxidant enzyme, superoxide dismutase. Copper works with iron to help the body form red blood cells. It also helps keep the blood vessels, nerves, immune system, and bones healthy.

❖ Basil leaves are an excellent source of iron, contains 3.17 mg/100 g of fresh leaves (about 26% of RDA). Iron, being a component of haemoglobin inside the red blood cells, determines the oxygen-carrying capacity of the blood.

❖ An important essential oil, eugenol has been found to have anti-inflammatory function by acting against the enzyme cycloxygenase (COX), which mediates inflammatory cascade in the body. This enzyme-inhibiting effect of the eugenol in basil makes it an important remedy for symptomatic relief in individuals with inflammatory health problems like rheumatoid arthritis, osteoarthritis, and inflammatory bowel conditions.

❖ Oil of basil has also been found to have anti-infective functions by inhibiting many pathogenic bacteria like *Staphylococcus, Enterococcus, Shigella* and *Pseudomonas.*

❖ Basil tea (basil water-brewed) helps relieve nausea and is thought to have mild anti-septic functions.

❖ The presence of remarkably high levels of beta-carotene, vitamin A, cryptoxanthin, lutein and zea-xanthin in basil, act as powerful antioxidants and protect against oxygen-derived free radicals and reactive oxygen species (ROS) that play a role in aging and various disease processes.

❖ Zeaxanthin is a powerful yellow flavonoid compound, that protects the eye by absorbing damaging blue light and reducing glare. Blue light can cause harmful oxidative stress in the eye.

Zeaxanthin protects cells and membranes by reducing harmful free radicals.

❖ The ashes of the roots are used as remedy for skin diseases. The seeds are laxative. The juice of leaves and flowers is used in case of cough.

❖ It is found effective in diabetes, cough and cold, ear infection, headache etc.

## Other Uses

❖ Fresh basil leaves add richness to vegetables and fruit salads

❖ *O. basilicum* is the most widely used in medicines, perfumes, cosmetics and liqueurs. Basil leaves are used to flavour any vegetable, poultry, or meat dish. The herb is also used in tomato and egg dishes, stews, soups, and salads.

❖ It is one of the principal ingredient of "pesto" a green sauce that is added to vegetables, fish, soups nd pasta dishes in Mediterranean cooking.

❖ Fresh or dried basil leaves are being used in the preparation of soups and dishes.

❖ In Asian countries a kind of flavour drink made of basil seeds is very popular.

## Home Remedies

❖ Basil leaves can be used in the treatment of fever and common cold. Chew some fresh basil leaves for relief from colds and fever.

❖ During the rainy season, when there is risk of malaria and dengue fever, try to consume tender leaves of basil after boiling it in water. This will help you to keep yourself safe from these kinds of fever. When suffering from acute fever, a decoction of the basil leaves boiled with powdered cardamom in one cup of water must be consumed several times a day. The juice of basil leaves can be used to bring down high temperature.

❖ In monsoon use of basil tea will give relief from cold and fever.

❖ Basil is also found to give relief in swine flu.

❖ Take 1 cup normal water mix 1/4 table spoon of carom seeds (ajwain) with 2 black pepper crushed to pieces with 4-5 holi basil leaves (tulsi leaves) and 1/2 table spoon ginger powder. Boil the mixture till it is half cup and drink it hot. Don't Drink Water for atleast 1 hour. This will give relief against cough and cold.

# CHAPTER 12

## Bhallataka: A Herb For Rheumatoid Arthritis

---

"Life is one percent what happens to you, and ninety-nine percent how you respond to it."

Shubhra Krishan

*Semecarpus anacardium* Linn (bhallataka) is one of the best versatile and most commonly used herbs as household remedy distributed in sub Himalayan region. The word Semecarpus is derived from Greek word Simeion meaning marking or tracing and carpus meaning nut. Anacardium means like cardium - heart shaped marking nut The nut is commonly known as 'marking nut' and in the vernacular as 'Ballataka' or 'Bhilwa'. Bhallataka has been freely used as medicine all over India since centuries. Bhallataka has the ability to penetrate deeply into the tissues and rejuvenate the body. Bhallataka was held in high esteem by ancient sages of *Ayurveda*. Maharshi Charak emphasized the Rasayana property of bhallataka and described 10 types of preparations with it. He considered bhallataka as the best drug to cure the *kapha* related diseases. Charak has categorized bhallataka has dipinaya as appetizer, bhedaniya-accumulation breaking herb, mutra sangrahaniya - antidiuretic, kusthaghna- antidermatosis. It is beneficial in failure of panis erection and sexual disability. Marany nut is a beautiful yet potentially deadly plant. Despite its darker side, this nut has been used for hundreds of years in traditional medicine. It has high priority and applicability in indigenous system of medicine. *Semecarpus anacardium* Linn. (Family: *Anacardiaceae*) is a plant well-known for its medicinal value in Ayurvedic and Siddha system of medicine. Earliet reference of bhallataka was found in paninisutra.

# Bhallataka Herb information

## 1. Nomenclature

Family Name: *Anacardiaceae*
Scientific Name: *Semecarpus anacardium* Linn
Sanskrit Name: Bhalataka, Arushkara, Shophakrut, Agnimukha marking nut, Common Names: Bhela, Bhilawa, Senkottai, Erimugi, Cashew
Common Name: Marking nut

## 2. Bio energies

Rasa: Ashaya, Madhura
Virya: Ushna, Laghu, Snigdha, Tikshna
Vipaka: Adhura
Karma: dipanapachana, bhedanam, jvaraghna, krimiaghna, kasahara, svasahara, kushtaghna, medhyam, kushtaghna, vajikarana, Vata*kapha*hara
Prabhava: The Ashtanga Hrdaya considers bhallataka fruit to be "…like fire in property"

## 3. Biomedical Action

Anti-cancer, anti-microbial.

## Habitat

Marany nut is indigenous to India, specifically the base of the Himalayas throughout the Coromandel region. It grows in these areas today at an elevation up to 1,000 m. Though bhallataka is found throughout India, it grows in abundance in the regions of Assam, Madhya Pradesh, Konkan and Gujarat. In the south India, the plant thrives in moist, deciduous Sub-Himalayan tract from the Bias eastwards, ascending in the outer hills up to 1,100 m. Assam, Khasia Hills, Chittagong, Central India and

the western Peninsula. Although some sources indicate that bhallataka
was brought to India from South America by the Portuguese, it is clearly
mentioned and described in both the Sushruta and Charak samhitas, texts
which antedate the Portuguese by more than millennia. *S. anacardium* is
now cultivated all over the world as medicinal plant. The plant is found
in abundance in Assam, Bihar, Bengal and Orissa, Chittagong, central
India and western peninsula of East Archipelago, Northern Australia.
food, in moist tropical forests, and in the subcontinent ranging from
the sub-Himalayas and Assam in the north, to the coast of Kerala in
the south.

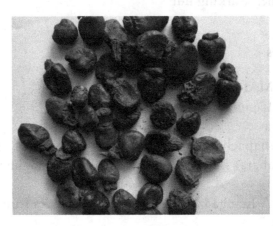

**Marany nut**

## Botanical Characters

Bhallataka is a medium-to-large size tree, 15–20 m in height. Leaves
simple, alternate, oblong, obovate, rounded at the apex 18-60 x 10-30cm.
with grey bark exfoliating in small irregular flakes; leaves simple alternate,
obviate – oblong, 17.5–60 cm long and 12–30 cm broad, rounded at the
apex. The flowers are greenish white, in panicles and appear with new
leaves in May and June, easily recognized by large leaves and the red
blaze exuding resin, which blackens on exposure. The nut is about 2.5
cm long, ovoid and smooth lustrous black. It is frequently found in drier
rather than damp localities. The fruit ripens from December to March
and are 2–3 cm broad. No specific soil affinity. It is a moderate shade
bearer, obliquely ovoid or oblong drupe, 2.5 to 3.8 cm long, compressed,

shining black when ripe, seated on an orange-coloured receptacle form of the disk, the base of the calyx and the extremity of the peduncle. The bark is grey in colour and exudes an irritant secretion on incising.

## Plant Part Used

Pericarp of the nut, a by-product of the cashew industry, gum, oil.

## Chemical Constituents

Bhallataka has been shown to contain the phenolic glucoside anacardoside and derivatives of anacardic acid that include a sub-class of compounds called the bhilawanols. Flavonoid constituents include semecarpuflavanone, semecarpetin, jeediflavone, galluflavanone and nallaflavanone. Bhallataka also contains an assortment of minerals, vitamins, amino acids and a fixed oil.

## Health Benefits

Bhallaraka is a powerpacked herb extensively used as medicine in *Ayurveda*.

❖ Bhallataka has long been considered an important remedy in the treatment of a variety of complaints including rheumatism, arthritis, neuritis, liver disorders and hemorrhoids, which is considered equal to mercury in action.

❖ It is also considered an important remedy in the treatment of asthma, and in skin diseases such as psoriasis, and was even highly valued in syphilis.

❖ It is one of the more effective remedies, along with yogaraja guggulu, in the treatment of rheumatoid arthritis.

❖ It is a specific tonic to male fertility as it increases semen production. As it helps to treat premature ejaculation and seminal leakage, it also treats incontinence and unrestrained urinary dribbles.

❖ It is very beneficial for vitiligo and other skin diseases affecting pigmentation.

❖ It strongly increases the appetite and treats conditions caused by low digestive fire; piles, diarrhoea, worms and colitis.

❖ It is used against dyspepsia, constipation, parasites, cough, asthma, leprosy, rheumatoid arthritis, sciatica, neuritis, diabetes, dysmenorrhea, infertility, weakness, fatigue, cancer, hepatocarcinoma (aflatoxin-induced).

❖ Its ability to clear *ama* helps to clear the srotas. Piles alleviates *vata* and *kapha* types of haemorrhoids. It goes directly to the root cause of the disease as it rectifies.

❖ Now a day's this plant found only in forest area because people are not properly aware with its importance or poisonous nature.

## Home Remedies

❖ One important Rasayana of ballataka recommended by Chakradatta called Amritabhallataka. To prepare this remedy boil 2.56 kg of ripe bhallataka fruits in 10 litres of water till reduced to 2.56 litres. Remove the fruits, add 10 litres of milk and 640 g ghee, boil on low heat until all the milk has evaporated and only the original volume of ghee remain(i.e. 640 g). Add An equal weight of gur mix thoroughly. Use after a week. The Chakradatta states that the dose is according to the "…digestive power," mentioning that this preparation is the "king of all Rasayanas," and may be used on an ongoing basis to promote strength and longevity microbial: An alcoholic extract of the dried nuts of S. anacardium showed a dose dependent in vitro antifungal activity against *Aspergillus fumigatus* and *Candida albicans*.

## Cautions

❖ The pericarp contains a variety of toxic principles that can precipitate a skin rash and renal failure if the dose is too large or if the remedy is prepared incorrectly. Prepared properly however bhallataka has been shown to be remarkably non-toxic and very safe.

# CHAPTER 13

## Bibhitaki: A Gift of Nature

---

The life of all living things is food; complexion, clarity, voice, growth and the intelligence all are established in food.

Charak

Bibhitaki is one of the oldest medicinal plant in India. Its botanical name is *Terminalia belerica* – Fructus. Bibhitaki is sanskrit word means "one who keeps you away from disease". It is a true gift of nature and possesses unique healing properties like very few other plants on this earth. Since thousand of years this herb is widely used as a remedy for the treatment of diseases affecting lungs, intestine and urinary tract. *T.belerica* is commonly found in Indian forests. Bibhitaki is a rejuvenative, beneficial for hair, throat, eyes and a laxative herb. Along with amalaki and haritaki, it is an incomparable ingredient in the Ayurvedic tonic triphala, where its function is, among others, to nurture and tone the tissues of the digestive system. It is known as a stomach and intestinal tonic and harmonizes all the processes of the digestive system.

**Bibhitaki Herb Information**

**1. Nomenclature**

Family name: *Combretaceae*
Scientific Name: *Terminalia belerica* – Fructus
Sanskrit Name: Bibhitaki
English Name: Beleric myrobalan

Common Name: Baheda, Beleric myrobalan, Bhomora, Bhomra, Bhaira, Beleric Myrobalan, Bahedam, Beheda, Bahera etc.

## 2. Bioenergestics

Rasa: Kashaya, Madhura
Guna: Dry, light
Virya: Ushna, laghu, ruksha
Vipaka: Madhura
Dosha effect: VPK=, aggravates *vata* in excess
Dhatu: Plasma, Muscle, Bone, Nerve
Srota: Digestive, Respiratory, Nervous, Excretory
Prabhava: Bibhitaki is called 'intimidating' because disease shrinks in the face of its power to heal.

## 3. Biomedical Properties

Expectorant, broncho-dilator, astringent, laxative, anthelmintic, astringent, anthelmintic, aperient, expectorant, sweet, anodyne, stypic, narcotic, ophthalmic, antipyretic, antiemetic and rejuvenating

## Habitat

Locally known as Baheda in India, has been used for centuries in the *Ayurveda*. The dried fruit used for medicinal purposes found growing wild throughout the Indian subcontinent, Sri lanka, and South East Asia. This is an important Ayurvedic tree found throughout the Indian forests and plains.

## Botanical Characters

Bibhitaki is a large deciduous tree with a buttressed trunk, thick brownish-grey bark covered with numerous fine longitudinal cracks, attaining a height of between 20 and 30m. The tree grows up to 1,200 m in elevation. Leaves 10-20cm long by 7-12 cm wide, elliptic, ovate.

Leaves when matured are glabrous and usually punctuate the upper side, midrib promonent. The leaves are crowded around the ends of the branches, Wood is yellowish grey, hard and course. alternately arranged, margins entire. Flowers – pale greenish yellow with offesive odour. The fruits are ovoid, grey, velvety, hard thick walled, 12- 25 mm in diameter. Nut is stony.

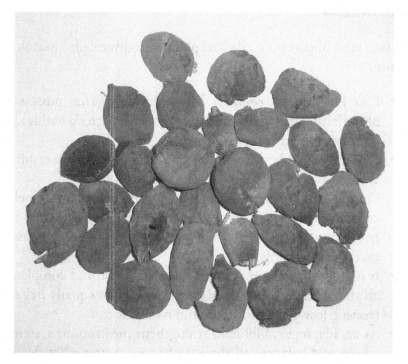

**Bibhitaki Fruits**

## Chemical Constituents

Detailed chemical analysis of bibhitaki indicate presence of following active principles. Triterpenoids (bellericoside, bellericanin, cardiac glycoside saponisn), sterols (beta-sitosterol) and tannin (gallic acid, ellagic acid). Active principles includes glucoside (bellericanin) gallo-tannic acid, colouring matter, resins and a greenish yellow oil. lignans(termilignan and thannilignan), flavone and anolignan. Tannins, ellargic acid, ethyl gallate, galloyl glucose and chebulaginic acid, phenyllemblin, mannitol, glucose, fructose and rhamnose.

## Plant Part Used: Fruits

## Health Benefits

*T. chebula* is an important medicinal plant with diverse pharmacological spectrum.

- ❖ Like Haritaki *(T. chebula),* Bibhitaki *(T. belerica)* possess anti-bacterial activity against many pathogenic bacteria and is a good remedy for many everyday illnesses.
- ❖ Bibhitaki is the best treatment for all sicknesses of the respiratory system.
- ❖ On one hand it soothes coughs, while on other hand it helps to expel phlegm from the lungs, during which it also nurtures them. In this way bibhitaki promotes the healing of wounds caused by excessive coughing.
- ❖ It is known as a stomach and intestinal tonic and complements all the processes of the digestive system. It is equally helpful in treating loss of appetite, gas, and parasites.
- ❖ As an adaptogen, bibhitaki strengthens the immune system as a whole, and balances all three doshas, no matter what the initial cause for the imbalance was.
- ❖ In *Ayurveda* the bibhitaki is classified as an expectorant. It is an integral part of well known laxative formulation triphala used in treatment of constipation and common cold.
- ❖ Results of one clinical trial, bibhitaki was found to have anti-asthmatic, anti-spasmodic, expectorant and anti-tussive activities.
- ❖ Oil extract from the seed pulp is used in leucoderma and alopecia. Modern investigations have proved the laxative activity of the oil.
- ❖ Bibhitaki is an antioxidant, it neutralizes the free radicals generated in the body thus reduces the aging process.
- ❖ When taken internally or applied externally to skin and hair, it exhibits remarkable nurturing effects. Especially good for

nurturing hair, it is used in cases of premature graying, and can also be used as a natural black dye.

❖ Present day scientific studies support the use of bibhitaki as a heart and liver tonic.

❖ It prevents the buildup of fat in both organs, and so diminishes the cause of many liver and heart diseases.

❖ Furthermore, in *Ayurveda* bibhitaki is used for treating infections of the eye, and increases eyesight.

❖ *T. belerica* is a valuable Rasayana, whose healing potential has yet to be fully realized. It will certainly going to get importance in 21ˢᵗ century.

❖ It helps in getting deep sleep and alleviates pain in *vata* disorders.

❖ It is best for treating alpha disorders, by removing mucous from the digestive tract helping in better absorption of nutrients by the body.

❖ Mature and dry fruit is constipating and is useful in diarrhoea.

❖ It is also useful in treating cardiac disorders, haemorrhage, leprosy, ulcers, urinary calculus, dyspepsia and general debility.

❖ The mature, dried fruit of bibhitaki is effective in the treatment of dysentery and intestinal parasites but should be taken along with purgatives such as Markandika (*Cassia angustifolia*) to counteract its constipating effects; the sun-dried unripe fruit however is gently aperient and can be used on its own.

❖ Bibhitaki is a good remedy in for vomiting in pregnancy.

❖ It is useful antilithic in gall bladder and urinary diseases, liquefying and expelling the stones.

❖ A decoction of the dried fruit may be taken internally and externally as an eyewash in the treatment of ophthalmological disorders.

❖ The kernel is typically removed before bibhitaki is used, and specifically stated to be narcotic used topically as an analgesic in the treatment of inflammation and pain, and internally in vomiting, bronchitis and colic.

❖ Other studies indicate that *bibhitaki* has retroviral actions in inhibiting the viral growth in leukemia patients, and yet another study indicates the strong inhibiting effect on the HIV virus.

❖ As a daily rejuvenating an preventative supplement bibhitaki is superb, especially for *kapha* body types. Bibhitaki reduces excess body water, fat, and slowly regenerates the body on a tissue level. For people prone to viral infections, or a history of leukemia in the family, Bibhitaki is a recommended daily supplement, alone or on the triphala formula.

## Home Remedies

❖ For severe cough and asthma the powder of the dried fruit may be taken with honey.
❖ Mix bibhitaki with saindhava (rock salt), pippali and buttermilk, in case of hoarseness.
❖ The fruit pulp mixed with ghee is covered with cow dung and heated in a fire, and held in the mouth to control coughing.

# CHAPTER 14

## Brahmi: #1 Herb For Cognitive Disorders

One of the most important features of modern medicine differentiating it from *Ayurveda* is the method of breaking complex phenomena into their component parts and dealing with each in isolation.

*Ayurveda*, a 5,000-year-old medical system, claims that Brahmi *(Bacopa monniera(L)* Wettst*)* is one of the best-known herbal medicine for improving learning, memory and recall. Brahmi is a Sanskrit word derived from "Lord Brahma" or "Brahman". Lord Brahma is the god of creation responsible for all of the creative forces in the world and Brahman is the Hindu name given to the universal consciousness. Brahmi literally means the energy of Brahma. Thus, Brahmi has a lot to offer to the medical world. Brahmi is an important medicinal plant that has been widely used therapeutically and is becoming increasingly popular in the west. According to *Ayurveda*, brahmi is characterized by lightness, peace and clarity and is good for all ages of people. Brahmi has been used for more than 3,000 years in traditional Indian medicine and is recognized the world over as a brain tonic to promote intellect and comprehension, rejuvenate the brain and boost the memory. People also take Brahmi to treat backache, hoarseness, mental illness, epilepsy, joint, and sexual performance problems in both men and women. It is also sometimes used as a "water pill." Brahmi is not gotu kola (*Centella asiatica*). Some reference books say that gotu kola is called Brahmi. A critical study of comparative photochemistry, pharmacology and therapeutic properties of these two drugs has proven that they are distinct. Both are esteemed Ayurvedic herbs. Brahmi was used specifically in mental diseases like insanity and epilepsy, while gotu kola (Mandukaparni) was used as a general brain tonic.

## Brahmi Herb Information

### 1. Nomencalture

*Family Name: Plantaginaceae*
*Scientific Name: Bacopa monniera(L)* Wettst
Sanskrit Name: Brahmi
English Name: Herb of Grace
Common Name: Andri, Bacopa, Bacopa monniera, Herb of Grace, Herpestis Herb, Herpestis monniera, Hysope d'Eau, Jalanimba, Jal-Brahmi, Jalnaveri, Nira-Brahmi, Moniera cuneifolia, Sambrani Chettu, Thyme-Leave Gratiola, Water Hyssop. Bacopa, Babies tear, Bacopa monnieri, Hespestis monniera, Nirbrahmi, Indian Pennywort, Jalanevari, water hyssop etc

### 2. Bioenergies

Rasa: Tikta
Guna: Laghu, sniddha
Virya: Ushna
Vipica: Katu
Prabhava: Medhya

### 3. Biomedical Action

Sedative, nervine, cardiotonic, anti-spasmodic, anti-convulsing, anti-inflammatory.y

### Habitat

Brahmi is found in humid and warmer parts of the world. It is found in marshy areas near streams and ponds throughout India especially in the north eastern regions. In India and the tropics it grows naturally in wet soil, shallow water, and marshes. It is found in Uttar Pradesh, Punjab, Haryana, Bihar, Bengal, Tamil Nadu, Kerala, and Karnataka. Brahmi is found in humid and warmer parts of the world hills of Himachal Pradesh. It is also widely grown in the Bandhavgarh National Park in India. Brahmi is an annual creeping plant found throughout India including the North Eastern region. The herb can be found at elevations from sea level to altitudes of 1,350 m(3,500 feet) and is easily cultivated, if adequate water is available. Flowers and fruit appear in summer and the entire plant is used medicinally.

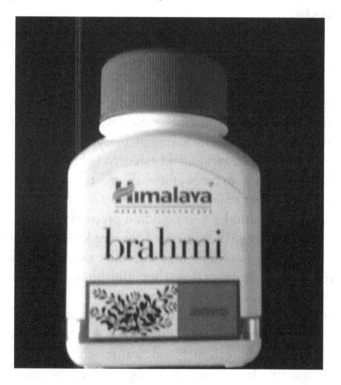

**Brahmi Product**

## Botanical characters

*Bacopa monniera,* is a small, creeping herb with numerous prostrate branches, each 10-30 cm long. succulent, rooting at the nodes, brahmi leaves are 1-2 X 0.4-1.0.cm in size. long petiole, oblong, sessile, and fleshy.

Small, tubular, five-petalled, white flowers develop in leaf terminals and can blossom over many months of the year. Small, dark seed set in a flat, oval capsule. Perennial ground cover to 10 cm high, with sprawling stems that may root.

## Plant Part Used

All parts

## Health Benefits

There are number of health benefits associated with this wonderful herb. some of them are

- ❖ Brahmi is a favorite brain tonic herb – it literally means "that which gives knowledge of Supreme Reality." Brahmi improves many brain functions including memory, learning ability, mental acuity and concentration, and can even help rejuvenate the brain cells. It's the #1 herb for cognitive disorders associated with aging!
- ❖ It is taken to get relief from stress and anxiety. According to the *Ayurveda,* Brahmi have antioxidant properties.
- ❖ Brahmi is highly recommended for employees who suffer from extreme stress, for students in difficult examination periods, for seniors to retain mental vitality, and for managers to increase their memory and concentration.
- ❖ Brahmi is used in *Ayurveda* for centuries. treatment of bronchitis, chronic cough, asthma, hoarseness, arthritis, rheumatism, backache, fluid retention, blood cleanser, chronic skin conditions, constipation, hair loss, fevers, digestive problems, depression, mental and physical fatigue and many more.
- ❖ It has been reported to reduce oxidation of fats in the blood stream, which is the risk factor for cardiovascular diseases. Brahmi is considered as the main rejuvenating herb for the nerve and brain.
- ❖ It is used to treat all sorts of skin problems like eczema, psoriasis, abscess and ulceration.

❖ A recent scientific study showed that brahmi has potent antioxidant properties, which is, no doubt, why it was also revered in India for strengthening the immune system, improving vitality and performance and promoting longevity. Along with the more familiar antioxidants, beta sitosterol, a powerful fatty acid in brahmi, acts to relieve many degenerative conditions.

❖ It is used in mental disorders, epilepsy, and hysteria. Brahmi also possess anticancer activity.

❖ It specifically enhances the quality of *pitta* and this directly influences the nature of consciousness. Nerves used to aid recovery from exhaustion, stress and debility with aggravation of *vata*. A specific herb for all conditions with a deficient majja dhatu. Consider using in Parkinson's disease, Alzheimer's, dementia, ADHD, Asperger's syndrome, autism, depression and drug addiction.

❖ Brahmi is very useful in skin conditions with an underlying nervous imbalance. It also benefits tension throughout the system helping to ease constipation from stress, relax muscle tightness and alleviate menstrual pain.

❖ It is commonly used to treat insomnia. It can cool the heat of cystitis and pain of dysuria by guiding *pitta* out of the urinary tract.

❖ In May 1996 the Royal Society of British Science called nitric oxide 'the marvel of the decade'. They found that the nitric oxide in brahmi has an extremely positive effect on learning and memory recall, as well as on blood circulation and the function of the liver, lungs and kidneys.

❖ As medicated oil it is a neuralgic in joint pain. Used as a head rub for headaches and to clear the mind. It is also used as a brain tonic to strengthen the memory and encourage hair growth.

❖ It has rare quality of lowering *vata* and *kapha* without raising *pitta*.

❖ Brahmi oil restores and preserves the memory. In India, it is given to the infants to boost memory power intelligence

## Other Uses

❖ Brahmi is rich in Vitamin C and can be used in the salads, soups and sandwiches.

# CHAPTER 15

## Ginger: Powerful Anti-inflammatory Herb

---

*Vata, pitta* & *kapha* **are physical doshas and Rajas** & **Tamas are mental doshas. Imbalance of** *vata, pitta* **or** *kapha* **causes physical ailments and imbalance of rajas or tamas creates mental illnesses.**

Charak

Ginger the rhizome of the plant *Zingiber officinale* Roscoe is a very popular spice and herbal medicine for 5,000 years. It is believed to be the native of South East Asia, India in particular. The plant's botanical name is thought to be derived from its Sanskrit name *singabera* which means "horn shaped," a physical characteristic of rhizome. Since long Ginger is used as medicine in Indian, Asian and Arabic culture. Ginger has been used to treat arthritis, diarhoaea, colic and heart conditions. Ginger's ability to combat a variety of diseases and conditions is due in part to its impact on excessive inflammation, which is a significant underlying cause of many illnesses. When something harmful or irritating affects a part of our body, there is a biological response to try to remove it, specifically acute inflammation, show that the body is trying to heal itself. Inflammation does not mean infection, even when an infection causes inflammation. Infection is caused by a bacterium, virus or fungus, while inflammation is the body's response to it.

**Ginger Herb Information**

**1. Nomenclature**

Family Name: *Liliaceae*
Scientific Name: *Zingiber officinale* Roscoe

Sanskrit Name: Lashuna, Rasona
English Name: Ginger
Common Name: Black ginger, Canton ginger, Cochin ginger, Common ginger, Garden ginger, Gingembre, Imber, Jamaican ginger.

## 2. Bioenergies

Rasa: Madhura, Tikta
Guna: Heavy, unctuous, penetrating
Virya: Ushna
Vipaka: Tikta
Dosha effect: VK-, P+
Dhatu: All tissues
Srota: Digestive, Respiratory, Circulatory, Reproductive, Mental

## 3. Bimedical Action

Anti-emetic, anti-inflammatory, anti-oxidant, anti-septic, anti-spasmodic, anti-viral, carminative, circulation-stimulating, detoxifying, diaphoretic, digestive, lymph-cleansing, mild laxative, perspiration-inducing, warming.

## Habitat

For centuries, ginger has been cultivated mostly in Asia. The ginger plant offers a large selection of uses from food to improving health. It is abundantly available throughout the tropical regions, like China and India. Chinese were the first in the world who realized the ecomical importance and started systematic cultivation of the ginger plant. It is a shade loving plant and grows well under partial shade, requires fertile soil, needs ample moisture, cool climate and heavy rainfall. It requires warm and humid climate. Recently, the ginger plant has been cultivated by people in tropical areas all over the world, particularly in Africa and Jamaica. Today, the top commercial producers of ginger include Jamaica, India, Fiji, Indonesia and Australia, Taiwan, Sierra Leone, Bangladesh, Philippines, Mauritius, Brazil, Costa Rica Ghana, Japan, Thailand.

Malaysia, Guatemala, and many pacific ocean islands. In India the crop occupies largest area in the state of Kerala, followed by Orissa and Meghalaya.

## Botanical Characters

The ginger plant is an erect perennial growing from 0.3 to 0.9 m in height. Ginger is a knotted, thick, beige underground stem, called a rhizome. The leaves are long, narrow, ribbed, and white or yellowish-

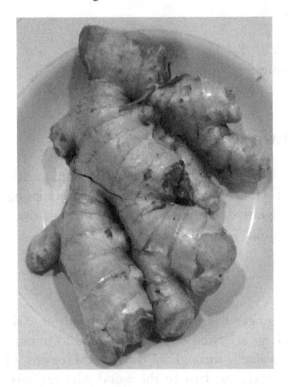

**Ginger rhizome**

green flowers. Ginger rarely flowers in cultivation. Rhizome branch with thick thumb like protrusions. Individual divisions of rhizome is called hands. Rhizomes are 7-15 cm long and 1 -1.5cm broad and laterally compressed. The flesh of the ginger rhizome can be yellow, white or red in colour, depending upon the variety. It is covered with a brownish skin that may either be thick or thin, depending upon whether the plant was harvested when it was mature or young. The ginger rhizome has a firm, yet striated texture and a taste that is aromatic, pungent and hot.

## Chemical Constiuents

The major active ingredients in ginger are terpenes which are similar to the chemical action of turpentine and an oleo-resin called ginger oil. These two, and other active ingredients confer antiseptic, lymph-cleansing, circulation-stimulating, and mild constipation relief qualities along with a potent perspiration-inducing action to ginger. The pungency of ginger is due to gingerol, an oily liquid consisting of homologous phenols. In the fresh ginger rhizome, the gingerols were identified as the major active components. Fresh ginger contains 80.9% moisture, 2.3% protein, 0.9% fat, 1.2% minerals, 2.4% fibre and 12.3% Carbohydrates. The powdered rhizome contains 3-6% fatty oil, 9% protein, 60-70% carbohydrates, 3-8% crude fiber, about 8% ash, 9-12% water and 2-3% volatile oil The minerals present in ginger are iron, calcium and phosphorous. It also contains vitamins such as thiamine, riboflavin, niacin and vitamin C. The composition varies with the type, variety, agronomic conditions, curing methods, drying and storage conditions.

## Health Benefits

There are endless health benefits of ginger.

❖ Some biochemical constituents of ginger inhibit the growth of colon bacteria like *Escherichia coli, Proteus* species, *Staphylococci, Streptococci and Salmonella*. It has been found that out of 29 different plant extracts tasted, ginger extract had the broadest range of anti-fungal activity.

❖ Ginger is very effective in preventing the symptoms of motion sickness, especially seasickness. In one clinical study ginger was compared with Dramamine, a over-the-counter and prescription drug for motion sickness. Ginger was found to be far superior reducing all symptoms associated with motion sickness including dizziness, nausea, vomiting, and cold sweating.

❖ Ginger contains powerful anti-inflammatory compounds called ginggerols. people with osteoarthritis, rheumatoid arthritis, gout experience reduction in their pain levels and improvements in their mobility when they consume ginger regularly.

❖ In one study ginger extract exhibited antitumor effects on colon cancer cells by suppressing their growth.

❖ A methanolic extract of dried rhizomes of ginger produced a significant reduction in lipid levels.

❖ Ginger possess an excellent carminative and intestinal spasmolytic properties. Ginger directly affect the gastrointestinal tract, helping to improve muscle tone and to prevent abnormally rapid and strong intestinal contractions.

❖ Ginger has been shown to possess anti-diabetic activity in a variety of animal studies. A study found that rats who received ginger juice significantly increased insulin level and fasting glucose levels. Treatment with *ginger* also produced other favorable effects in diabetic rats, including decreases in serum cholesterol, triglycerides, and blood pressure.

❖ Anti-vomiting properties of ginger is useful in controlling nausea and vomiting of pregnancy, even the most severe form.

❖ Modern scientific research has revealed that ginger possesses many therapeutic properties including antioxidant effects, an ability to inhibit the formation of inflammatory compounds, and direct anti-inflammatory effects.

❖ Ginger has also been recommended as remedy for arthritis, fevers, headaches, toothaches, coughs, bronchitis, to lower cholesterol and aid in preventing internal blood clots.

❖ It is a warming remedy, ideal for boosting the blood circulation, lowering high blood pressure and keeping the blood thin in higher doses. Ginger is anti-viral and makes a warming cold and flu remedy.

❖ Ginger root is a medicinal herb used primarily for the treatment of dyspepsia (discomfort after eating), this includes the symptoms of bloating, heartburn, flatulence, and nausea.

❖ It is used to ease menstrual cramps.

❖ Ginger may also be taken orally as a herbal remedy to prevent or relieve nausea resulting from chemotherapy, radiation, pregnancy, and surgery.

❖ If a person has exercised too much or suffers from arthritis or rheumatism, ginger has been known to ease inflammation of the joints and muscle tissue. Due to its tremendous circulation-increasing qualities, ginger is thought to improve the complexion. It has reduced nervousness, eased tendonitis, and helped sore throats return to normal.

❖ Studies demonstrate that ginger can lower cholesterol levels by reducing cholesterol absorption in the blood and liver. It may also aid in preventing internal blood clots.

❖ Recent studies may confirm that ginger directly affects the gastrointestinal tract, helping to improve muscle tone and to prevent abnormally rapid and strong intestinal contractions

## Home Remedies

❖ In case of cold and flu, consume ginger several times a day. It will help detoxify your body in a natural manner, which will make you feel better and speed up the healing process.

❖ Boil one teaspoon of ginger powder or two teaspoons of freshly grated ginger in two cups of water and inhale the steam to alleviate congestion and other symptoms associated with common colds.

❖ To treat the arthritis pain, apply warm ginger paste with turmeric to the affected area twice a day. Also, include raw or cooked ginger in your diet.

❖ To improve digestion, try to eat ginger after any large meal. Ginger can also help alleviate the various symptoms of food poisoning.

# CHAPTER 16

## Gotu kola: The Plant of Regenerative Therapy

---

**I think that age as a number is not nearly as important as health. You can be in poor health and be pretty miserable at 40 or 50. If you're in good health, you can enjoy things into your 80s.**

Bob Barker

Gotu Kola, also known as Indian Pennywort is one of the most widely used and important Ayurvedic herbs on the market today. *Centella asiatica Linn* is known as longevity herb and used widely in India and Nepal as part of the traditional Ayurvedic medicine. It is also called 'Mandukaparni' as its leaf appears as a standing frog from its backside. The plant's name coins from the Greek words hydor, meaning water, and cotyle, meaning cup. Gotu kola has been used to treat many health conditions for thousands of years in India, China, and Indonesia. It has been called "miracle elixirs of life". It is believed to develop the crown chakra, the energy center at the top of the head and to balance the right and left hemispheres of the brain, the shape of which resemble to leaf. It was the life history of the renowned Chinese herbalist Professor Li Chung Yun, who lived to the age of 256 years which made the western world aware of the true value of this wonderful herb for longevity. A legendary saying, in reference to gotu kola was: 'two leaves a day, keeps old age away'. Gotu kola is not the same as kola nut (*Cola nitida*). Gotu kola neither have caffeine nor is a stimulant. It was Sri Lankans who noticed that elephants renowned for their longevity, ate on the leaves of this plant. Thus the leaves became known as a promoter of long life. It is said to fortify the immune system, both cleansing and feeding it and to strengthen the adrenals. Gotu Kola is a rejuvenative nervine plant recommended for nervous disorders, including epilepsy, senility and premature aging.

## Gotu kola Herb Information

### 1. Nomenclature

Family Name: *Apiceae (Umbelliferae)*
Scientific Name: *Centella asiatica Linn*
Sanskrit Name: Brahmamanduki, Brahmi, Bheda, Bhekaparni, Bheki, Brahmamanduki, Darduchhada, Divya, Mahaushadhi, Mandukaprnika, Manduki, Mutthil, Supriya, Tvasthi
English Name: Gotu kola
Common Name: Jal Brahmi, Mandūka Parni, Indian pennywort, Pennywort. Bemgsag, Brahma-Manduki, Gotukola, Khulakhudi, Mandookaparni etc.
Synonym: *Hydrocotyle asiatica L, Hydrocotyle pallida DC*

### 2. Bioenergies

Rasa: Tikta, Kasaya, Madhura
Guna: Laghu, Sara
Virya: Sīta
Vipaka: Madhura
Dosha effects: VPK =
Dhatus: Blood, Marrow and Nerve
Prabhava: Medhya

### 3. Biomedical Action

Sedative, nervine, cardiotonic, anti-spasmodic, anti-convulsing, anti-inflammatory

## Habitat

Plant grows abundantly in shady, moist, or marshy areas and river banks. It is distributed widely in many parts of the world. *Centella asiatica* found throughout tropical and sub-tropical regions of India up to an altitude of 600m. The plant has been reported to occur also at high altitudes of 1550m in Sikkim and 1200m in Mount Abu (Rajasthan). The plant is indigenous to South-East Asia, India, Sri Lanka, parts of China, the Western South Sea Islands, Madagascar, South Africa, South East USA, Mexico, Venezuela, Columbia and Eastern South America. It is indigenous to tropics of both hemispheres including Asia, Africa, Australia, Central America, South America and Southern United States. Although usually gathered wild, gotu kola can be cultivated from seed in spring.

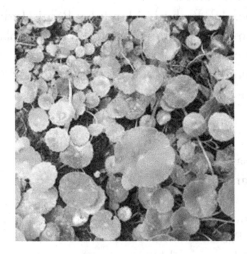

**Gotu kola Plant**

## Botanical Characters

*Centella asiatica (L.)* is a small prostrate, faintly aromatic, perennial, creeper herb, attains height up to 15cm (6 in), width 2-5cm. Stem is glabrous, striated. The stems root at the nodes. *Centella asiatica* flourishes extensively in shady, marshy, damp and wet places such as paddy fields, river forming a dense carpet. Flowers are so small which are reddish and rising from the center and often hidden underneath leaves that, generally, the flower is not noticed at all. It is only under a microscope that the flower's beauty is seen. The leaves, 1-3 from each node of stems, Petioles are erect and long ; 2- 6cm long and 1.5-5cm wide, renniform, sheathing leaf base, crenate margins. Size of leaves can depend on climate, season, soil structure, fertility and growing position: whether in sun or shade. Flowers are in fascicled umbels, each umbel consisting of 3-4 white to purple or pink flowers, flowering occurs in the month of April-June, blooms in summer. Fruits are borne throughout the growing season in approx. 5 cm long, oblong, globular in shape and strongly thickened pericarp. The crop matures in three months and the whole plant including roots is harvested manually.

## Chemical Constituents

Scientific studies have proved the presence variety of different biochemical components in gotu kola, which reflects the importance of this herb in current system of medicine. *C. asiatica* is reported to have below mentioned types of chemicals. Triterpenoids, volatile and fatty acids, alkaloids, glycosides, flavonoids, tannins, saponins, phytosterols, amino acids, sugars, volatile oils. There are three main chemical constituents in the plant. The first is asiaticoside, which is a triterpene glycoside and classified as an antibiotic. They are probably responsible for the wound healing and vascular effects. The second constituent is a pair of chemicals, brahmoside and brahminoside, which are saponin glycosides. These are diuretic in nature and have a slightly sedative action in large doses. Finally, there is a glycoside that is a powerful anti-inflammatory agent. The plant also contains vitamin K, magnesium, calcium and sodium.

## Plant Parts Used

Whole plant (leaves, seeds, fruits)

## Health Benefits

*C. acitika* has wide spectrum of medical application.

❖ Charak described the importance of gotu kola as anti-aging medicinal plant, apart from its role in treating tuberculosis.

❖ Extract of this plant accelerates cicatrisation and grafting of wound. Asiaticoside promotes fibroblasts proliferation and extracellular matrix synthesis in wound healing. In Ayurvedic medicine it is used for chronic and stubborn skin conditions such as eczema and psoriasis. Gotu kola helps to reduce scaring.

❖ A double-blind, placebo-controlled study on the effects of gotu kola *(C. asiatica)* on healthy persons. Results of preliminary findings suggest that gotu kola has anxiolytic activity in humans as revealed by the ASR. It remains to be seen whether this herb has therapeutic efficacy in the treatment of anxiety syndromes.

❖ In China gotu kola is used for dysentery and summer diarrhoea, vomiting, jaundice and scabies, hansen's disease, (leprosy), nosebleeds, tonsillitis, fractures, measles, tuberculosis, urinary difficulties, as a endocrine tonic and as an 'adaptogen'.

❖ Triterpenoids -a group of compounds found in gotu kola are believed ease anxiety, according to a study.

❖ Results of studies indicate that gotu kola may stimulate circulation and help fight varicose veins and venous insufficiency.

❖ Ointments containing gotu kola are used to treat wounds and other skin problems.

❖ Gotu kola has been used as a tonic for purification of blood and for promoting healthy skin. It has also been used to aid in restful sleep, treat skin inflammations, as a treatment for high blood pressure and as a mild diuretic.

❖ The leaves of this plant have been used around the world for centuries to treat, cancer, skin disorders, arthritis, hemorrhoids, and tuberculosis. In recent years, it has become popular in the west as a nerve tonic to promote relaxation and to enhance memory.

❖ The herbs calming properties make it well suited for overcoming insomnia and making one calm for yoga and meditative practices. It is commonly used to rebuild energy reserves improve memory and treat fatigue, both mental and physical.

❖ The plant has been referred to as "food for the brain". This oriental herb has demonstrated mild tranquilizing, anti-anxiety and anti-stress effects, as well as improving mental functions such as concentration and memory.

❖ Significant results obtained in healing of skin, other connective tissues, lymph tissues, blood vessels, and mucous membranes. Researchers have found that it contains several glycosides that exhibit wound healing and anti-inflammatory activities and that asiaticosides stimulate the formation of lipids and proteins necessary for healthy skin.

❖ It affects various stages of tissue development, including the process of replacing skin after sores or ulcers, the synthesis of collagen, the stimulation of hair and nail growth, and support for the repair of cartilage. It has been used in the treatment of second and third degree burns, and has been shown to decrease healing time and reduce scar tissue formation.

❖ Recent studies show that it also has a positive effect on the circulatory system. It appears to improve the flow of blood throughout the body by strengthening the veins and capillaries. It has been shown to be particularly useful for people who are inactive or confined to bed due to illness.

❖ The herb has been used successfully to treat phlebitis (inflammation of the veins), varicose veins, as well as leg cramps, swelling of the legs, and "heaviness" or tingling in the legs. In modern health care it has been used for venous insufficiency, localized inflammation and infection, and post-surgery recovery.

## Cautions

❖ Although side effects are rare, some people taking gotu kola may experience upset stomach, headache, and drowsiness. Because gotu kola can make your skin more sensitive to the sun, it's important to limit your sun exposure and use sunscreen while taking it.

❖ Medical experts advise against using gotu kola if you have a history of squamous cell carcinoma, basal cell skin cancer, or melanoma. People with liver disease should also avoid gotu kola.

❖ Gotu kola is not recommended during pregnancy

❖ Itching aggravation, headache or temporary loss of consciousness in large doses.

# CHAPTER 17

## Guduchi: A Divine Herb

"Through knowing death we can hold a beacon of love for every moment that has just passed, for every friend who has lost a friend, for every child who has lost a parent, for every parent who has lost a child; for any suffering anywhere."

Sebastian Pole

Guduchi (*Tinospora cordifolia* willd) Hook. F. & Thomson is large deciduous climbing shrub which is classified in the family *Menispermaceae*. Guduchi also known as amrit is one of the most valued herbs in the *Ayurveda*. In sanskrit it is known as gudduchika while hindi it is called giloya which refers to the heavenly elixir. According to vedic mythos, when the ancient gods churned the prehistoric ocean, an ambrosial nectar was created that would confer immortality on any who swallowed it. The nectar was named 'amrit', a sanskrit word that means 'divine nectar' or "imperishable." Recent studies support guduchi's role as adaptogens – a potent herb that increases the body's resistance to stress, anxiety, and illness. Guduchi is a sanskrit name means the one which protects our body. In India guduchi has been used for thousands of years but it is only just beginning to be available in the West. It is one of the most versatile rejuvenating herbs, it promotes longevity. It has been mentioned in various ancient Ayurvedic texts such as Charak Samhita, Sushruta Samhita, and Ashtang Hridaya as Rasayana. It is the best Rasayana for rejuvenating the body and getting rid of deep rooted imbalances. In fact, it is so full of life that it can grow without any soil or water. The herb supports the normal function of the immune system by maintaining optimal levels of white blood cells like macrophages

# Guduchi Herb Information

## 1. Nomenclature

Family Name: *Menispermaceae*
Scientific Name: *Tinospora cordifolia* (willd) Hook. F. & Thomson
Sanskrit Name: Guduchika, Amritavalli, Guduchi, Madhuparni, Amrita, Kundalini, Vatsadaani
English Name: Amrit, Heart-leaved Moonseed
Common Name: Gucha, Giloe, Gilo, Amrita bali.

## 2. Bio-energetics

Rasa: Tikta, Kashaya
Guna: Laghu
Virya: Ushna
Vipaka: Madhura
Dosha: VPK +
Karma: Balya, Dipana, Rasayana, Sangrahi, Tridoshashamaka, Raktashodhaka, Jvaraghna
Dhatu: Plasma, Blood, Muscle, Fat, Nerve, Reproductive

## 3. Biomedical Action

Cholagogue, detoxicant, immune modulator, anti-inflammatory, diuretic, anthelminthic, nervine tonic.

## Habitat

Guduchi is a climbing deciduous shrub which usually takes support of bigger trees. This plant can be mostly seen on top of other trees particularly mango and neem trees. Those growing up neem tree is considered to be the best. Guduchi is a parasitic plant, it draws total nourishment from the host plant. The synergy between two bitter plants increases the efficacy of guduchi. The plant is widely distributed in

India, extending from the Himalayas down to the southern part of peninsular India ascending to an altitude of 300m (1,000ft). It is found in China, Bangladesh, Pakistan, Myanmar and Sri lanka. The plant is also reported from South East Asian countries such as Malaysia, Indonesia, and Thailand etc. Plant prefers to grow in wide range of soil, acid to alkaline and it needs moderate moisture level.

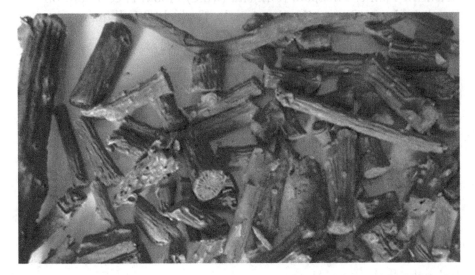

**Guduchi stem**

## Botanical Characters

Guduchi is a large deciduous corky climber with grooved stem. The leaves are heart shaped with pointed leaf tip, dark green, glabrous 5 – 10 cm long. The flowers are unisexual (male and female flowers are separate), small, yellow or greenish yellow. The stem is rather succulent with long filiform fleshy aerial roots from the branches. The thickness of the stem is generally about 1 cm in diameter but sometimes it can be as thick as 6 cm. The bark is creamy white to grey, The flowers are small and yellow or greenish yellow, the male flowers are clustered and female are usually solitary. The drupes are ovoid, glossy, succulent, red and pea sized. Flowers grow during the summer and a fruits during the winter. The fruits are called drupes, which are found in clusters, single seeded. The seeds are curved. Fruits look like bunch of red cherries. Fruits turn red when ripened. Arial roots, are found in the Himalayas and in many parts of south India.

## Chemical Constituents

Guduchi has got a variety of pharmacologically and medicinally useful chemical constituents, which are being utilized in the field of *Ayurveda* Scientists have isolated and identified number of chemical compounds from diferent parts of guduchi, which are classified as 1. steroids, 2. alkaloids, 3. glycosides, 4. diterpenoid lactones, 5. aliphatic compounds,6. polysaccharides. In adition to this T. cordifoliia leaves of this plant are tinosporone, tinosporic acid, cordifolisides A to E, syringen, berberine, giloin, gilenin, crude giloininand, arabinogalactan polysaccharide, picrotene, bergenin, gilosterol, tinosporol, tinosporidine, sitosterol, cordifol, heptacosanol, octacosonal, tinosporide, columbin, chasmanthin, palmarin, palmatosides C and F, amritosides, cordioside, tinosponone, ecdysterone, makisterone A, hydroxyecdysone, magnoflorine, tembetarine, syringine, glucan polysaccharide, syringine apiosylglycoside, isocolumbin, palmatine etc. The drug is reported to possess one fifth of the analgesic effect of sodium salicylate, which is commonly used in allopathic medicine as an analgesic and an antipyretic.

## Plant Part Used

Roots, Stem, Leaves and Sattva

## Health Benefits

Guduchi has wide spread uses in maintaining health of an individual.

❖ Guduchi clears *pitta* toxin and uric acid accumulated in blood vessels. It also removes *ama* toxin from the body. Removal of toxin will give some relief to patients of arthritis, gout, and inflammatory joints.

❖ Guduchi is diuretic in action. It assists to expel urinary stone from the kidney. It is also helpful in the management of urinary tract infections.

❖ It is effective against asthma, jaundice, skin infections, anorexia, diarrhoea, diabetes, leprosy.

❖ Guduchi is considered as a liver protector. It is helpful in treating liver damage, viral hepatitis and alcohol, medical or chemical poisoning of liver. It is useful in the management of fibrosis and regenerating liver tissue.

❖ It is recommended as adjuvant therapy to cancer patients who are undergoing chemotherapy.

❖ Guduchi is one and only Ayurvedic medicine which can bind and remove mercury, lead, heavy metals; once the toxin is flushed out from the body, intelligence is reestablished.

❖ Results of the laboratory experiment indicate that with administration of guduchi root extract in diabetic rats resulted in noticeable control of serum cholesterol. The results have been noted to be at par with standard drugs used to control cholesterol.

❖ Ulcers can be a result of excessive acid secretion in stomach, which damages the stomach walls. Generally, the stomach wall lining is affected regularly but, the stomach repairs it by making a new wall lining. But, if the stomach is not able to fully heal its wall lining, then the result is formation of ulcers. These ulcers have been controlled to an appreciable level by guduchi extracts.

❖ It is classified under the category of Rasayana, which accords to longevity, enhances memory, better complexion, voice energy and luster of skin thus bestows youth.

❖ All auto-immune diseases causing inflammation. Applicable in degenerative diseases such as cancer, AIDS and arthritis as it boosts the immune system..

❖ Superlative and inflammatory skin conditions such as eczema, psoriasis, Useful when there is high tejas and *pitta* that has burnt immune protecting ojas away resulting in inflammatory skin conditions. Skin problems from excessive alcohol, recreational drug and pharmaceutical drug use may indicate the use of guduch.

❖ Guduchi is the #1 Rasayana (rejuvenative herb) in *Ayurveda* because it can really reverse aging, support the immune system and detoxify. It has the ability of making a person look youthful. Ultimately PMS were statistically reduced by administering guduchi extracts.

❖ *T.cordifolia* (7.82% in 5 ml of syrup) is a best remedy for children suffering from upper respiratory tract infections.

❖ It is a calming herb for *vata* disorders.

❖ Extact of guduchi has been tested in women suffering with post-menopausal syndrome which can have symptoms such as breast discomfort, nausea and fluid retention. These symptoms and ultimately PMS were statistically reduced by administering guduchi extracts. The herb helps increase the efficacy of the protective white blood cells (WBC) and builds up the body's own defense mechanism. It inhibits bacterial growth and increases the body's immunity by enhancing the functioning of protective cells and macrophages.

❖ The aqueous extract of *Tinospora cordifolia* significantly reduced the serum cholesterol and maintained the HDL cholesterol level to basic value

❖ Dry barks of *T.cordifolia* has anti-spasmodic, anti-pyretic, anti-allergic and anti-leprotic properties.

❖ The aqueous extract of *T.cordifolia* root has anti-oxidant property.

❖ Guduchi has been reported to treat throat cancer.

❖ *Tinospora cordifolia* stem is bitter, stomachic, stimulates bile secretion, enriches the blood and cures jaundice, urinary disease and upper respiratory tract infection.

❖ The aqueous extract of stem is useful in skin diseases. The root and stem extract with combination of other drugs are prescribed as an anti-dote to snake bite and scorpion sting.

## Cautions

❖ People with diabetes should take this herb under medical supervision.

❖ Its usage in pregnancy sould be monitored under strict medical supervision.

# CHAPTER 18

## Guggulu: A Weight Reducing Herb

"Science of yoga and *Ayurveda* is subtler than the science of medicine, because science of medicine is often victim of statistical manipulation."

Amit Ray

Guggal (guggulu in Sanskrit) is a highly valued botanical medicine used in *Ayurveda*. Guggul is the yellowish resin extracted from the mukul tree (*Commiphora mukul* (Stocks) Hook or *Commiphora wightii (Arn.) Bhandari*). Widely used for thousands of years in *Ayurveda* and other traditional medicines for a variety of health conditions and as incense in holy ceremonies; Recently guggul has attracted the attention of west possibly because of its ability to treat high cholesterol and obesity. The classical text Charak Samhita described in detail the usefulness of this herb in the treatment of obesity and other disorders of fat including coating and obstruction. Guggul resin is produced more abundantly and is stronger in potency during the season of autumn; hence it must be collected in autumn. Freshly collected guggulu has a weight increasing quality, whereas Purana guggul (guggul which is at least one year old) has an weight reducing quality.

### 1. Nomenclature

Family Name: *Burseraceae*
Scientific Name: *Commiphora mukul* (Stocks) Hook or *Commiphora wightii (Arn.) Bhandari*

Sanskrut name: Guggulu, Dhurta, Divya, Durga, Guggalu, Jatala, Jatayu etc.

Engish Name: Guggal

Common Name: Indian Bdellium Gum, Guggulipid, Gum Guggul, Salaitree Gugulipid, Moql, Moqle-arzagi, Gugal, Gugali, Gugar, Guggul, Mukul.

## 2. Bio energies

Rasa: Tikta, Kashaya
Guna: Laghu, rukha
Virya: Ushna
Vipaka: Katu
Prabhav: Rasayana
Dosha effect: VKP=

## 3. Biomedical Action

Alterative, anti-inflammatory, (powerful), antipyretic, antiseptic, anti-spasmodic, anti-suppurative, aperient, aphrodisiac, astringent, bitter, carminative, demulcent, diaphoretic, disinfectant, diuretic, emmenagogue, enhances phagocytosis, immunostimulant, (increases leukocytes), stimulating expectorant, stomachic, thyroid stimulant, uterine stimulant.

## Habitat

Guggul is believed to have originated in Central Asia or Northern Africa. But, today, it is cultivated in India as well mainly for medicinal purposes. Guggulu plant is a highly tolerant plant as it can survive in areas where there is hardly any water. The plant is grown throughout the north India. The herb has been playing a major role in the traditional medicine of India.

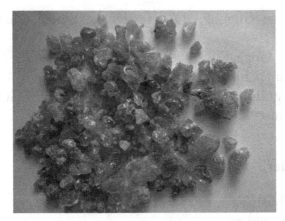

**Guggal Gum**

## Botanical Characters

Guggul is a resin, which is secreted by a small to medium sized, thorny mukul myrrh tree called *Commiphora mukul*. The shrub reaches a maximum height of 1.2 to 1.6m (4 to 6 feet) and bears thorns on its branches. The leaves are small similar to those of neem. The flowers are red and the fruit is oval in shape and pulpy in nature. The plant belongs to the Burseraceae family. The bark of the tree is used in Ayurvedic medicines and it is thin like paper. The branches are filled with thorns and the leaves trifoliate. The gum, called "guggul" or "gum guggulu," is tapped from the stem of the plant, and the fragrant yellow resin latex solidifies as it oozes out. Excessive production of the gum eventually kills the plant. *C. mukul* is synonymous with *C. wightii* and is in the same genus as *C. myrrha*.

## Plant Part Used

Exudate from stem

## Chemical Constituents

The gum contains minerals, resin, volatile oils, sterols, ferulates, flavones, sterones, and other chemical constituents. The ketonic steroid compounds known as guggulsterones. These compounds have been shown to provide the cholesterol- and triglyceride-lowering actions noted for guggulu.

Several pharmacologically active components have been identified in the plant, including guggulsterone (E- and Z-stereoisomers) and gugulipid, both found in the ethyl acetate extract of the plant. Studies have shown that the guggulsterones are antagonist ligands for the bile acid farnesoid X receptor, which is activated by bile salts, thus reducing cholesterol.

## Health Benefits

Since ancient times guggal has been used in treating health problems

- ❖ Guggul significantly lowers serum triglycerides and total cholesterol as well as LDL and VLDL cholesterols (the bad cholesterols).
- ❖ Encouraged by Ayurvedic description of this drug in lowering cholesterol, scientists have conducted clinical trials to test the efficacy of this herb in lipid metabolism and for weight reduction. The research resulted into the development of natural cholesterol substance. That is safer and more effective than many conventional cholesterol lowering drugs.
- ❖ At the same time, it raises levels of HDL cholesterol (the good cholesterol). As antioxidants, guggulsterones keep LDL cholesterol from oxidizing, an action which protects against atherosclerosis.
- ❖ Guggul has also been shown to reduce the stickiness of platelets, another effect that lowers the risk of coronary artery disease.
- ❖ One double-blind trial found guggul extract similar to the drug clofibrate for lowering cholesterol levels. Other clinical trials in India (using 1,500 mg of extract per day) have confirmed guggul extracts improve lipid levels in humans.

The major Ayurvedic medicines having *C. wightii* as an important ingredient are following.

**Types of Guggulu**

1. **Amrita Guggulu:** This formulation treats all the sixteen types of skin diseases viz; urticaria, enlargement of liver, leprosy, malignant jaundice, tubercular leprosy, loss of appetite, fistula-in-ano, catarrh in the nose, and abdominal ailments. It reduces hyperuricaemia and maintains proper uric acid levels in blood. These herbs are specifically effective against gout, vitiated air in the blood besides other uses such as acid-peptic disorders, piles, ulcers, diabetes, loss of digestive heat, arthritis, edema etc.

2. **Yograj Guggulu:** It used for old and high *vata* related conditions of the joints and muscles (Rheumatoid arthritis). It maintains healthy metabolism and removes toxins from the system. It rejuvenates and strengthens the neuromuscular systems. It is used in case of painful thigh, osteoporosis, bone density, gout, siffness nervous disease, epilepsy, cardiac lesions, anaemia, tumour, pain in chest etc.

3. **Punarnava Guggulu:** It is a combination of trikatu, triphala and guggal. It can remove deep seated *kapha* from the tissues. This guggal preparation is powerful detoxifying and rejuvenating in action. It supports the healthy elimination of liquids and helps maintain balance of the water element within the body. It is used for sciatica pain and stiffness of thigh, leg and lumbar region; colic pain in urogenital system and arthritis. Edema, Gout, Hyperuricemia (an excess of uric acid in the blood creating inflammatory and painful swelling of joint, limbs, and appendages), purine metabolism, gouty conditions, water retention.

4. **Kishore Guggulu:** Its main ingredients are guduchi, trikatu, triphala ang guggal. This is also powerful detoxifying and rejuvenating combination aimed primarily at removing deep-seated *pitta* from the tissues This preparation is especially balancing for *pitta*, particularly when it is disturbing the musculoskeletal system. It also acts to nourish and strengthen the system, supporting the overall health and proper function of the joints, the muscles, and the connective tissue.

5. **Shuddha Guggul:** Guggul is purified in cow's milk in order to remove toxic substances and render the guggulu easily

absorbable. *Ayurveda* specifies Shodhana (purification) as one of the important procedures before oral administration of guggul. This type of guggulu is used in lowering cholesterol, triglyceride, *vata* related disorders.

6. **Triphala Guggulu:** Triphala Guggulu is a well-balanced mixture of two very effective herbs described in *Ayurveda*. While Triphala is one of the most effective bowel cleansers, Guggul works as an effective defense agent for the body. This mixture is being used in India for various curative purposes for more than 4,000 years. Benefits in fatigue, constipation, indigestion, mal-absorption, diabetes, low metabolism, high cholesterol, high blood pressure, sinusitis, allergies, sinus congestion, rheumatism, arthritis, hemorrhoids, toxemia, hyperglycemia, general debility, brittle nails, inflammation, flatulence, dullness in skin, myopia, headaches.

## Dosage

Dosage recommendations for guggul are usually based on guggulsterones concentration in the extract. A typical dosage of guggulsterones is 25 mg three times per day. Most extracts can be taken daily for 12 to 24 weeks for lowering high cholesterol and/or triglycerides.

## Home Remedies

❖ Take 1 to 2 teaspoonfuls of guggulu powder 2 to 3 times a day with hot hot or lukewarm water or milk, ir reduces the temperature and improves thyroid functions.
❖ Take 25 mg of guggal powder daily for 12 to 24 weeks to purify blood and reduce skin diseases
❖ To stay away from acne guggal is the best recommended medicine for teenagers.

## Cautions

Although the use of guggul in therapeutic doses appears to be safe and non-toxic, the following precautions are advised.

❖ Guggul is considered an emenogogue (an agent that promotes the menstrual discharge) and a uterine stimulant, and should not be used during pregnancy.

❖ In addition, caution is recommended with patients currently on prescribed medications for cardiovascular disease. Due to the diuretic action of this herb the following drug interactions are possible: increased risk of toxicity with anti-inflammatory analgesics.

❖ Finally, during the course of using guggulu one should avoid the following: foods that are sour or bitter in taste, alcohol, excessive exercise, physical and mental strain, anger, and exposure to direct sunlight.

❖ High doses of guggul may cause allergies itching and shortness of breath.

❖ If you are a thyroid patient before taking guggul you must consult a physician.

It won't be surprised if, in near future, guggal turns out to be the possible panacea for most of the chronic ailments particularly afflicting human race.

# CHAPTER 19

## Haritaki: A Digestive Tonic

**The great thing about** *Ayurveda* **is that its treatments always yield side benefits, not side effects**

Shubhra Krishnan

Haritaki *(Terminalia chebula)* is one of the most important medicinal plants used in most ayurvedic recipes in the treatment of several diseases. Because of number of pharmacological properties, haritaki is extensively used in *Ayurveda*, homeopathy, unani and siddha system of medicine. In Sanskrit "Hara" is also the name of Lord Shiva, thus reflecting the sacred nature and elevated position of the plant. The revered Charak declared the fruit of this south Asian tree to be a powerful rejuvenator, and the best in fighting off sicknesses. The plant is also named as Pathya, owing to its beneficial effect for the channels (patha) of the body. Haritaki is that fruit which removes all diseases from the body and brings a luster and shine to the skin. Legend has it that haritaki tree produced from a drop of nectar (amrita) fell to the earth. Accordingly, in Tibetan medical philosophy, it is called as the "king of all medicinal plants". Haritaki is most widely known as a component of the Ayurvedic preparation triphala, but exhibits noteworthy healing effects both individually and in combination with other herbs. Though haritaki is a common drug, it is observed the drug is not used in the proper way. Actually the entire fruit is to be used unless otherwise specialized to obtain the optimum therapeutic efficacy of the drug.

## Haritaki Herb Information

### 1. Nomenclature

Family Name: *Combretaceae*
Scientific Name: *Terminalia chebula* – Fructus *(retaceae)*
Sanskrit Name: Haritaki, Abhaya
English Name:: Chebulic myrobalan
Common name: Chebulic myrobalan, Harde, Hara
Synonyms: Haritaki, Abhaya, Shiva, Bhishagwara, Rudrapriya, Harade, Himaja, Pilo Hardae, Chhoti Har, Halda, Har, Haraa, Haraaraa, Harad, Harara, Harash, Harb, Harda, Harir, Haritaki, Haritali, Harra, Pile Hara etc

### 2. Bioenergetics

Rasa: All but salty, mainly kashaya, bitter
Guna: Light, dry
Virya: Ushna
Vipaka: Madhura
Dosha effect: VPK=
Dhatu: All tissues
Srota: Digestive, Excretory, Nervous, Respiratory

### 3. Biomedical Action

Laxative, astringent, anthelmintic, nervine, expectorant, tonic

### Habitat

*T. chebula* is capable of growing in a variety of soils, clay as well as shady The trees may grow at places up to a height of about 2,000 m from the sea level, and in areas with an annual rainfall 100-150 cm and temperature 0-17° C. In India, it is quite prevalent all over Northern India reaching in the outer Himalayas up to an altitude of 2,000 m, from Ravi to West Bengal. It's occurrence is particularly abundant in the Kangra Valley of the Himalayas, Punjab, Assam, Bihar, Karnataka, Western Ghats, Tamil Nadu, Orissa, Kerala, Andra Pradesh, Uttar Prdesh, West Bengl, Madhya Pradesh, and Maharashtra. T. chebula, though, is a native of Asia, but also found in Nepal, Sri Lanka, Myanmar, Bangladesh, Egypt, Iran and Turkey and also in Pakistan and Yunnan, Tibet, Guangdong, Guangxi province of China.

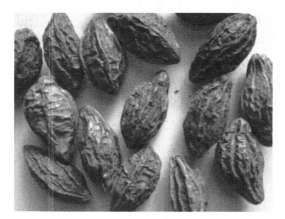

**Haritaki Fruits**

## Botanical Characters

The large deciduous haritaki tree grows at an altitude of 1,800 m attaining 25 – 30 m height, 1.5 – 2.5 m diameter. It has round crown and spreading branches. Branches, young leaves and leaf buds are covered with soft shining coloured hair. Leaves 10 – 20 cm long, ovate, rounded acute apex. The flowers are dull white, bisexual with a strong unplesant smell. Fruit is a drupe, 2-4 cm long and 1.3-1.5 cm broad, hard and yellowish green in colour, each fruit has a single seed. It has five lines or five ribs on the outer skin. Bark 6 mm thick, dark brown with some longitudinal cracks. Flowering in May to September and fruiting in July to December. Fruit is green when unripe and yellowish grey when ripe

## Chemical Constituents

*T. chebula* contains tannins up to 30%, chebulic acid 3-5%, chebulinic acid 30 %, tannic acid 20-40%, ellagic acid, 2,4-chebulyi–β-D-glucoyranose, gallic acid, ethyl gallate, terchebin, anthraquinone, flavonoids like luteolin, rutins, and quercetin etc. Some of the other minor constituents were polyphenols such as corilagin, galloyl glucose, punicalagin. Besides, fructose, amino acids, succinic acid, beta sitosterol, resin and purgative principle of anthraquinone are also present. Flavonol, glycosides, triterpenoids, phenolic compounds were also isolated. Twelve fatty acids were isolated from *T. chebula* of which palmitic acid, linoleic acid and oleic acid were main constituents.

## Plant Part Used

Fruits

## Health Benefits

*T. chebula* is extensively used since anciet times against number of disesases.

- ❖ *Terminalia chebula* is a true digestive tonic. It ignites the fire of digestive tract and so helps the body to digest and absorb total nutrients.
- ❖ Haritaki is also used in combination with bibhitaki and amalaki to prepare a formulation called Triphala. This medicine is widely used as anti aging formula and also as laxative.
- ❖ Haritaki is also believed to have powerful effect on intestinal parasites such as *Amoeba giardia* and many others parasites.
- ❖ It is used in the preparation of medicines for the treatment of infectious diseases like leucorrhoea, chronic ulcers, pyorrhea and other types of fungal infections of the skin.
- ❖ It is a strong laxative, and is used to cleanse the digestive system by moving waste thoroughly.
- ❖ *T. chebula* is also believed to improve intelligence and alertness in a person.

❖ In the *Ayurveda* an ancient healing system haritaki is used to treat all sorts of eye disorders – inflammation, conjunctivitis. Not only is it recommended for eye infections due to its antibacterial properties, but it also strengthen and improves eyesight.

❖ In addition haritaki nurtures and improves both the liver and the spleen in their function. These processes lead to the rejuvenation of the whole body, and prove haritaki to be an invaluable Rasayana of Ayurvedic medicine.

❖ Present scientific knowledge indicate that the gallic acids contained in haritaki exhibit antibacterial as well as antifungal axtion which might be playing a key role in control of diseases.

❖ It is also used for increasing the immunity of the body. Haritaki is used in the treatment of mouth ulcers, stomatitis, asthma, cough, gastroenteritis, skin diseases, leprosy etc.

❖ It is also used for treatment of intermittent fever, rheumatic pain and fever, wounds and arthritis. Haritaki is one of the best herbs for treatment of *vata* dosha; it is used as a natural remedy for flatulence; indigestion etc.

❖ It reduces lipid deposits in the blood and liver.

❖ Furthermore, haritaki is used to treat respiratory illness, and is effective in cases of bronchitis and chronic asthma. Also used as a purgative in ayurvedic treatments. It is also used as a tonic and expectorant.

❖ Haritaki is called as the mother of human being. As a mother never does bad for her progeny similarly haritaki never does bad for the health of a fellow. It benefits a fellow in all aspects

❖ It sends accumulated *vata* downwards and helps to clear wheezing, weak voice and asthma.

❖ Another avantage of haritaki is it heals ulcers. Mouth ulcer, stomach ulcer, gets healed. And the oxygen level in the blood drastically increases

## Home Remedies

❖ To achieve laxative action of Haritaki, adult dose of powder is 3 to 6 g. and for children, the dose of Haritaki is 0.5 to 1 g. to be taken with lukewarm water once a day on an empty stomach. It is preferably taken early in the morning or minimum three hours after dinner. Haritaki is useful in constipation, haemorrhoids, stomatitis, hyperacidity and associated gastrointestinal disorders.

## Cautions

- ❖ No side or toxic effect of Haritaki is reported with its recommended dose. Clinical studies have also shown no adverse effect in patients treated with Haritaki alone or with formulations.
- ❖ Avoid taking dry diet and a diet with higher fibre content and liquids is advisable for the patient.
- ❖ It should not be prescribed to pregnant women. It is safe for the baby if the nursing mother is taking this medication.
- ❖ The astringent and dry property of Haritaki may induce nausea in sensitive individuals. This may be masked by consuming it in tablet form or by preparing its decoction and adding jiggery to it.
- ❖ Dose of Haritaki as a laxative varies from person to person according to their constitution, digestive power and bowel habit. Administration of Haritaki should be stopped if the desired effect is not achieved.

# CHAPTER 20

## Long Pepper (Pippali): An Anti-diabetic Agent

"We can't talk about our own health without understanding our place in our environment, because in order to fulfill our potential we have to live in the context of our surroundings. We have to know our place in the ecosystem of which we are a part, and this means living 'consciously'; being aware of nature and how it affects us and how we, in turn, affect nature

Sebastian Pole

Long pepper is known as *pippali* in India. The word pepper itself is a sanskrit word for long pepper. Apart from its use as a popular spice, long pepper also have several medicinal properties. It is helpful in various health problems. Documented evidence of pippali as multipurpose drug was first decribed in Charak Samhita. where it is listed alongwith *Rasayana*. *It is* mentioned for the treatment of cough, pumonary respiratory distress, gastro-intestinal disorders, cough, pulmonary tuberculosis etc. In Ayurvedic medicine long pepper is used for enhancing digestion and metabolism. It is in combination with dried ginger and black pepper to form famous Ayurvedic preparation "*trikatu*", which is very effective in regulating cholesterol level. It helps to prevent obesity. Pippali has a folklore reputation as an aphrodisiac, and is believed to improve vitality. Long pepper has a long history of use throughout the Mediterranean, Africa, India and Indonesia, to which the plant is native. Hippocrates was the first person to write about health benefits of long pepper. The fruits are harvested around January while still green and unripe, as they are most pungent at this stage and of high medicinal value.

## Pippali Herb Information

### 1. Nomenclature

Family Name: *Piperaceae*
Scientific Name: *Piper longum Linn., P. pepuloides, P. officinarum*
Sanskrit Name: Pipalika, *Magadhi*, Granthika
English Name: Long Pepper
Common Name: Piparamula, Pippali, Bengal Pepper, Indonesian Long Pepper, Java Pepper, Lada Panjong,

### 2. Bio energetics

Rasa: Katu
Guna: Laghu (Light), Ruksa, snigdha (unctuous), tikshna (sharp)
Virya: Ushna
Vipaka: Madhur, Katu
Dosha: KV+, P -
Karma: Dipana, *Kapha*hara, Pachana, Ruchya, Vatahara, Vatanulomana, shoolaprashamana

### 3. Biomedical Action

Antibacterial, Astringent, Carminative, Cholagogue, Diaphoretic/sudorific Immenagogue, Vermifuge, aphrodisiac, febrifuge, expectorant, uterine stimulant, diuretic, emmenagogue.

### Habitat

India is a leading producer, consumer and exporter of long pepper in the world. The herb is a slender, creeping, annual plant that is native to hot parts of the country, although it is found abundantly in the wild as well. While Kerala and Karnataka account for most of the production of black pepper in the country (around 92%), it is extensively cultivated in West Bengal as well. The herb grows well in the hot and humid parts of sub- continent. Long pepper is a native of Indo-Malaya region. It is found growing wild in the tropical rain forests of India, Nepal, Indonesia, Malaysia, Sri Lanka, Rio, Timor and the Philippines. Indian long pepper is mostly derived from the wild plants. The herb also grows wild in Bhutan, Myanmar and elsewhere.

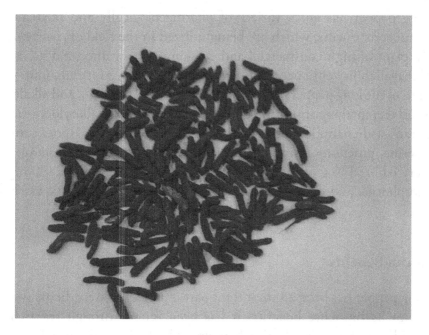

**Long pepper Fruits**

## Botanical Characters

Long Pepper or *Piper Longum* Linn is a flowering vine that is usually dried and used as a spice and as seasoning. Plant flourishes well in organic matter rich fertile, well-drained loamy soils. Laterite soils rich in organic matter content with good moisture holding capacity are also suitable. A slender aromatic climber with perennial woody roots; stems creeping, jointed; leaves 5-9 cm long, 3-5 cm wide, ovate, cordate with broad rounded lobes at base, subacute, entire, glabrous; spike cylindrical pedunculate, axillary or extra axillary, green at first turning to yellow later. Flowers minute, unisexual, male larger and are 2.5-7.5cm long and

slender, female 1.3-2.5 cm long and 4-5mm. diam.; fruits small, dark red
when ripe, oid, yellowish orange, sunk in fleshy spike.

## Chemical Constituents

Long pepper has got a variety of pharmacologically and medicinally
useful constituents, which are being utilized in the field of *Ayurveda*. It
is a plant of high commercial and economic importance and its use as
a bioavailability enhancer can be explored in various formulations. The
fruits of the long pepper plant contain 1 % volatile oil, resin, and alkaloids,
piperine, piperlongumine, piperlonguminine, and N-isobutyldeca-trans-
2-trans-4-dienamide along with a terpenoid substance. Roots contain
piperine, piperlongumine (or piplartine), and dihydrostigmasterol. For
every edible 100 g of the fruit, there is 1230 mg of calcium, 190 mg of
phosphorus, and 62 mg of iron. The fruit also contains some essential
oils.

## Health Benefits

Long pepper has been an important part of our age old medicine system
due to its immense benefits. It has been found through research to
provide the following health benefits. The fruits and roots both are
attributed with numerous medicinal benefits.

- ❖ Diabetes is becoming a serious concern in today's medical world,
  and to our discomfort, India has a large number of diabetes
  patients and very soon India is going to become diabetes capital
  of the world. Long pepper could prove to be an effective anti-
  diabetic remedy. Experimentally it is observed that long pepper
  significantly brings down blood glucose levels. Hence, it is used
  in the preparation of cinnamon tea, which is taken by diabetic
  patients to reduce blood sugar levels in type 2 diabetes.
- ❖ India being tropical country, our warm weather allow easy
  proliferation of bacteria. Bacteria are responsible for a large
  number of health problems. Both the root and fruit of long pepper
  possess anti-bacterial properties against number of bacteria and
  are also known to display anti-amoebic activity.

❖ Long pepper is known to exhibit hepato-protective activity on liver and hence prescribed long pepper to be taken with boiled milk to patients of Jaundice and to those afflicted with liver.

❖ The roots and fruits have a bitter and hot sharp taste and are recommended in palsy, night blindness, gout and lumbago problems, diseases of respiratory tract viz.; cough, bronchitis, asthma, etc. As counter-irritant and analgesic, when applied locally for muscular pains and inflammation.

❖ It is used as snuff in coma and drowsiness and internally as carminative ; as sedative in insomnia and epilepsy.

❖ Fruits are capable of increasing intellect and memory power.

❖ Pepper is also used as general tonic and in obstruction of bile duct, gall bladder, dysentery and leprosy.

❖ Long pepper is used as a nerve depressant and also has antagonistic effects on electro-shock and chemo-shock seizures for muscular spasms.

❖ Long pepper also has antibacterial properties in addition to having tonic, stimulant, analgesic and carminative properties.

❖ One of the other major health benefits of long pepper is that it helps in increasing the appetite. It also helps in driving out gas from intestines. Problems such as stomach aches and tumors can also be cured with the help of long pepper.

## Vardhaman Pippali

Adharya Charaka has described this special technique of consuming long pepper in increasing order to alleviate lungs disorder and many more diseses. On the first day of treatment, take one half cup of water and one half cup of milk and one long pepper (pippali) and boil until water evaporates, and drink the milk, on the second and successive days, add one additional pippali until the total number reaches the number of seven, nine or eleven.(i.e. two pippali on 2nd day, three on 3rd day, four on 4th day ....and so on). Duration of treatment is decided as per patient's need. Then reduce the amount taken each day by one until the amount of one long pepper is again reached. This cycle should be repeated for three months. This is the slow method of rebuilding the lung tissue. This technique without demaging the lungs, increases their energy in a way that persists for a long period of time. If the pippali is consumed in the above fashion, it is said to promote bulk and induces enormous strength, allievates hoarseness of voice and other vocal disorders and makes the voice strong, bold. Prolongs the life span and enables one to live a disease free life.

## Other Uses

❖ Apart from many health benefits, long pepper is also useful in a number of other ways. Long pepper is the key ingredient in many pepper spray products as a self defense mechanism. The main advantage that long peppers have over other traditional fruits is that they are simple to use, versatile, affordable, and have instantaneous effects. common cold, pharyngitis, laryngitis, bronchitis.

❖ It is always beneficial to include a little bit of long pepper into your diet. Not only do this pepper adds flavour to the food but also ensures that you will stay healthy and fit.

## Home Remedies

❖ Pippali powder is recommended for acute and chronic cough due to respiratory catarrh, respiratory allergy, asthma, sneezing, hiccough, nasal discharge, fever, poor appetite. The adult dose of the pippali is 1 - 3 g and the children's dose is 125 mg to 250 mg, two or three times a day, mixed with honey or warm water. Honey is the best vehicle for consuming Pippali powder. Jaggery or liquorice root powder may be used in place of honey, if the cough is dry, irritating and persistent. Warm water should be taken after consuming the medicine to facilitate its swallowing and fast absorption.

## Cautions

❖ No toxic effect or adverse reaction is reported with recommended.

❖ *Long pepper* should be used with caution in the first trimester of pregnancy. However, it is safe for the baby if a nursing mother is taking this medication.

# CHAPTER 21

## Rasona: A Boon For High Cholesterol

---

**"If we doctors threw all our medicines into the sea, it would be that much better for our patients and that much worse for the fishes."**

Supreme Court Justice Oliver Wendel Holmes, MD

$G$*arlic (Allium sativum)* is a member of the family *Liliaceae* has been widely recognized as valuable remedy for number of diseases. The botanical name, *Allium* may have originated from the Celtic word 'all' meaning pungent and the word *sativum* from the Latin word 'sative', meaning sown from the seeds. Rasona is a Sanskrit word means 'lacking a taste', derived from rasa meaning 'taste' and una meaning 'lacking', as except sour taste it contain all six tastes. Rasona, well known as Lasuna among Indians. Garlic is practically grown throughout the world, it is believed that garlic appears to have originated in central Asia then spread to China, and the Mediterranean region before moving west to Central and Southern Europe, Northern Africa (Egypt) and Mexico. Historical records show its medicinal use about 5,000 years ago, and for at least 3,000 years, it is a part of Chinese medicine. It is a boon for conditions like high cholesterol, high blood pressure and even deposition of the toxins inside the body. In addition of its reputation as a healthy food, garlic's anti- bacterial, anti-viral, anti-fungal, and antioxidant properties have also been demonstrated. The Egyptians, Babylonians, Greeks, and Romans used garlic for healing purposes. In 1858, Louis Pasteur noticed garlic's antibacterial activity, and in England it was used as an antiseptic to prevent gangrene during World War I and World War II. Garlic's current principal medicinal uses are to prevent and treat cardiovascular disease by lowering blood pressure and cholesterol, as an antimicrobial, and as a preventive agent for cancer. The active constituents are several complex sulfur-containing compounds that are rapidly absorbed, transformed and metabolized. The delicious bulbs of this annual are a veritable herbal panacea.

## Rasona Herb Information

### 1. Nonencalture

Family name: *Liliaceae*
Scientific Name: *Allium sativum – Bulbus*
Sanskrit Name: Lashuna, Rasona,
English Name: Garlic, Lashun
Common Name: Garlic, Lashun, Lasan

### 2. Bioenergetics

Rasa (taste) Tikta, madhura
Virya: Ushna
Vipaka ; Tikta
Guna (quality) Heavy, unctuous, penetrating
Dosha effects: VK-, P+
Dhatu: All tissues
Srota: Digestive, respiratory, circulatory, reproductive,
Karma: Balya, Caksusya, Dipana, Hrdya, *Kapha*hara, Medhya, Raktadosahara, Vatahara, Vrsya, Varnya, *Pitta*dusanakara, Bhagnasandhanakara, Rasayana, Jantughna, Kanthya, Asthi, Mamsa Sandhankzar

### 3. Biomedical Action

Carminative, vermifuge, vasodilator, expectorant, anti-cholesterol, anti-bacterial/fungal/ viral, anti-oxidant, fibrinolytic,

## Habitat

Garlic is believed to have first grown in central asia, from where its cultivation and use spread to the rest of the world. It is now commonly cultivated in the Mediterranean region, Egypt, Kenya, India, China, Philippines, and Brazil. It grows well in areas with cool and dry climates. The plant grows erect as an annual or biennial plant.

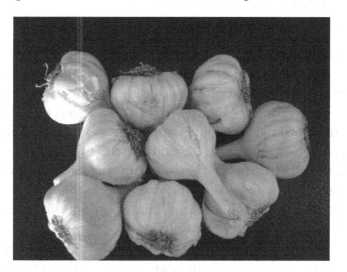

**Rasona Bulbs**

## Botanical Characters

The leaves are long 200 – 1,000 mm in length, alternate; there is one leaf per node along the stem. Leaves are growing only at the base of the plant. Leaf blade is linear, very narrow with more or less parallel sides. Flower petal colour is green to brown, white or pink to red, flower petal length 3-5 mm. The inflorescence is an umbel type. Because of short axis it appears that all flowers originate from the same point. The fruit is a capsule type. The bulb which is the only eaten part is of compound nature, consisting of many bulblets, technically known as cloves grouped together between membranous structure and enclosed within white thin skin, which hold them together in a sac.

**Plant Parts Used**

Fruits

**Health Benefits**

Garlic has number of health benefits.

- ❖ It modifies pulse, modulates the rhythm of the heart and relieves symptoms of high blood pressure and dizziness.
- ❖ Garlic helps to lower serum lipids, and breaks down cholesterol that might have accumulated in the blood vessels. This way it helps in restoring elasticity to the arteries, thus preventing heart attacks. Garlic is a popular supplement as a healthy choice among people looking to increase cardiovascular wellness.
- ❖ It directly benefits the heart by reducing *kapha* and *am*a in the rasa, rakta and meda dhatus and this has the effect of lowering blood cholesterol and reducing clotting; potential use in thrombosis and varicose veins.
- ❖ It enhances the body's immunity as well as directly removing pathogens. It can be both prophylactic and therapeutic for many infections. Garlic supports immune function in patients with AIDS.
- ❖ *Helicobacter pylori* is responsible for causing stomach ulcers. Galic is found to inhibit the growth of this bacteria.
- ❖ As a circulatory stimulant it warms the whole body. This regulatory effect on the circulation is further demonstrated by either lowering or raising blood pressure depending on the condition it balances, restores and regulates.
- ❖ Garlic selectively kills microorganisms that might be harmful for the body while also keeping normal flora of intestinal tract. It stimulates the secretion of digestive juices and cures inflammations of the digestive tract as well. This is a unique mechanism of repair of intestistal lining.
- ❖ Garlic extracts have been tested and found to be effective as aphrodisiac, and cures impotency when taken regularly.

❖ As Garlic Powder is well known to improve the blood circulation to all parts of body including skin; it is a recommended dietary supplement for skin diseases. Garlic Powder is one of the best dietary supplements to increase libido.

❖ Garlic powder is a good healer of fractured bone so it is a recommended dietary supplement for fractured bones, weak bones and in osteoporosis.

❖ Garlic Powder is a supporter of digestive system in all aspects. It is a well known fact that piles are the resultant of disturbed digestive system. so it is a natural remedy for piles.

❖ As Garlic Powder nourishes the every part of body it is one of the best *Ayurveda* supplement to increases physical strength

❖ Presence of sulphur, is rejuvenative for the respiratory system. This is the reason garlic powder is a recommended as dietary supplement for asthma and other respiratory system problems.

❖ The body nourishing characteristic of garlic powder makes it a good supplement for weight gain. If you want to use garlic to improve your health, the best way is by ingesting at least one clove a day.

❖ Rasona is extensively used in the treatment of rheumatoid arthritis, sciatica, lumbago, back pain and cervical spondylitis.

❖ It is also recommended in the treatment of leprosy, diseases of nervous system, infections by bacteria and viruses, intestinal worms etc.

❖ Garlic has an astounding effect on diabetes since one of its extracts (allicin) acts as anti-diabetic agent. It also lowers blood glucose levels.

❖ Garlic's anti-inflammatory properties make it particularly effective against arthritis, lumbago, and rheumatism.

❖ Garlic extracts were tested and found to reduce the absorption of lead and cadmium (which are toxic, heavy metals) in internal organs such as liver and the kidney, thus reducing the effect of toxic heavy metal poisoning.

❖ Garlic is highly nutritious. 28 g of garlic will provide 23% daily requirement of manganese, 17% of vitamin B 6, 15% of vitamin C, 6% of selenium. In addition it contains calcium, copper, potassium, iron, phosphorus and provide 42 calories.

❖ It boosts immune system. In one study it is proved that daily garlic supplement reduce the incidence of cold by 63 %. The average length of cold was also reduced by 70 %.

❖ In one study garlic supplementation have a significant impact in reducing blood pressure in people with history of high blood pressure.

❖ Garlic supplement can reduce total cholesterol and LDL. However it has got no effect on triglyceride level and HDL.

❖ We know that oxidative damage due to free radicals is the root cause of aging and diseases. Garlic contains antioxidants that protect against cell damage. The combined action of reduction in cholesterol and antioxidant may help prevent Alzheimer and brain diseases.

❖ Modern science has shown that Garlic is a powerful antibiotic, broad-spectrum rather than targeted. The body does not appear to build up resistance to the garlic, so its positive health benefits continue over time.

❖ Garlic could help people to live long.

❖ Garlic acts as an effective antiseptic while also relieving the patient of pain from the wound.

**Home Remedy**

❖ Instill medicated oil in the affected ear drop by drop by tilting the head to opposite side and retain it for about 30 minutes by plugging the ear with cotton swab. Repeat the process for other ear if affected. Instillation of oil in the ears can be done twice daily for 2-3 days. Medicated mustard oil is prepared by taking slightly crushed fresh 5-6 cloves in 20 ml mustard oil and and heating in low fire for 5-10 minutes till garlic become brown. Filter through cloth and use when ever needed. Recommended for earaches.

# Cautions

❖ Garlic may be used safely in pregnancy and breast-feeding. However, consumption by breast-feeding mothers may impact the infant's behavior during breast-feeding, causing prolonged attachment to the breast and increased sucking.

❖ People allergic to garlic may develop a rash from touching or eating the herb. Consult your practitioner before using garlic if you are pregnant

❖ Avoid large amounts of garlic if you are taking aspirin or other drugs that thin the blood

❖ Avoid garlic for 10 days prior to operative surgery. There may be a positive interaction with statins by increasing the cholesterol lowering effects and monitoring is advised.

# CHAPTER 22

## Shatavari: A Female Fertility Herb

---

The disease is simple and the remedy is equally simple. It is your mind only that makes you insecure and unhappy. Anticipation makes you insecure, memory – unhappy. Stop misusing your mind and all will be well with you. You need not set it right – it will set itself right – it will set itself right as soon as you give up all concern with the past and the future and live entirely in the now.

*Nisargadatta Maharaj*

Shatavari (*Asparagus racemosus Wild*) is powerful rejuvenating herbs in Ayurvedic medicine. It is commonly used in India for conditions affecting the female reproductive system, including the mood swings and irritation associated with premenstrual syndrome, as well as menopausal hot flashes. The Sanskrit word, shatavari, comes from the word *shat* (meaning one hundred) and *avari*(meaning marriage; sometimes translated as "she who possesses 100 husbands," Shatavari also has a reputation as a fertility-enhancing plant that improves the health of both male and female reproductive tissues; and as a support for the digestive system, especially in cases of excess *pitta*. This support is not only for the young woman, but also for the middle aged and elder lady, to help a woman gracefully transition through the natural phases of life, including menopause. Shatavari roots used as a drug acting on all tissues as a powerful anabolic. It is good for eyes, muscles, reproductive organs, increases milk secretion and helps to regain vigour and vitality. Charak Samhita written by Charak and Ashtang Hridaya written by Vagbhatta, the two main texts on Ayurvedic medicines, lists *Asparagus racemosus* as part of the formulas to treat disorders affecting women's health.

# Shatavari Herb Information

## 1. Nomenclature

Family Name: *Liliaceae*
Botanical Name: *Asparagus racemosus Wild*
English Name: Indian Asparagus
Sanskrit Name: Shatavari
Other Names: *Asparagus racemosus,* Satavar, Shatamooli, Shatavari, Shatawari, Challan gadda, Sadawari Kannada: Majjigegade

## 2. Bioenergies

Rasa: Madhur, katu
Virya: shita
Vipaka: Madhur
Effects on Dosh: VPK +ve

## 3. Biomedical Action

Mucilaginous, anti-diarrheic, refrigerant, diuretic, anti-dysenteric, nutritive, tonic, demulcent, galactagogue, aphrodisiac, antispasmodic, galactogogue, astringent, antidysentiric, laxative, anticancer, anti-inflammatory, blood purifier, antitubercular, antiepileptic.

## Habitat

*Asparagus racemosus* (Satavar, Shatavari, or Shatamull) is a species of Asparagus common throughout Sri Lanka, India and the Himalayas. It grows 1 – 2 m tall and prefers to take root in gravelly, rocky soils high up in piedmont plains, at 1,300–1,400 m elevation. It was botanically described in 1799. Due to its multiple uses, the demand for *Asparagus racemosus* is constantly on the rise. Due to destructive harvesting, combined with habitat destruction, and deforestation, the plant is now considered 'endangered' in its natural habitat.

**Botanical Characters**

Shatavari is a climbing undershrub with woody terete stems and recurved and rarely straight spines. Young stems very delicate, brittle, and smooth; leaves reduced to minute chaffy scales. Fruits subglobose berries, purplish black when ripe. Seeds 3-6, globose, or angled having brittle and hard testa. The tuberous succulent roots are 30 cms to a meter or more in length. Flowers are white, smooth tapering at both ends.

**Chemical Constituents**

The chemical ingredients in the shatavari plant, including steroidal saponins, isoflavones, asparagamine (an alkaloid substance similar to aspirin), and polysaccharides, make this plant a natural chemical source. The following active constituents are present is shatavari plant.

The major active constituents of *A. racemosus* are steroidal saponins (Shatavarins I–IV) that are present in the roots. Shatavarin IV is a glycoside of sarsasapogenin having two molecules of rhamnose and one molecule of glucose. Other active compounds such asquercetin, rutin (2.5% dry basis) and hyperoside are found in the flowers and fruits; while diosgenin and quercetin-3 glucuronide are present in the leaves.

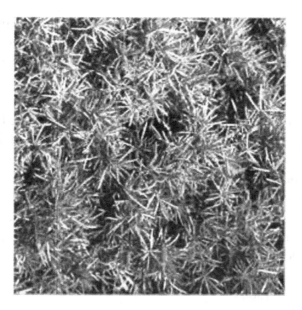

**Shatawari Roots**

## Plant Parts Used

Flashy Roots

## Health Benefits

Shatavari has many health benefits

- ❖ Shatavari is often prescribed in India to improve the production of breast milk in nursing mothers, though there has been relatively little scientific research to verify its effectiveness in this area.
- ❖ Shatavari has nourishing, soothing, and cooling properties that help with many conditions in which the body and mind are overheated, depleted, or out of balance — including heartburn, indigestion, diarrhoea, inflammation of the urinary tract, and irritable bowel syndrome.
- ❖ Scientists have also discovered that shatavari helps the immune system recover more quickly from exposure to toxins by protecting

blood-producing cells in the bone marrow and by enhancing the production of immune-regulating messenger molecules.

❖ Shatavari is used in *Ayurveda* to balance *pitta* and *vata,* but can increase *kapha* due to its heavy nature. Its bitter and sweet taste has a cooling effect on the system, and its unctuous (oily), building nature makes it a great support for anyone looking for a nourishing, grounding effect. These combined qualities make it a Rasayana (rejuvenative) for the reproductive system (particularly female), the digestive system (particularly when *pitta* is involved), and for the blood. Shatavari Powder is the main rejuvenative herb for women. It nourishes female reproductive organs thus enhancing female fertility. It tones and nourishes the female reproductive organs.

❖ Shatavari helps to relieve pains and controls blood loss during menstruation.

❖ Shatavari is a support for menopausal symptoms such as hot flashes. shatavari powder also promotes maternal health.

❖ It is mild aphrodisiac in nature.

❖ It is also useful in pre-menstrual symptoms thus gives relief in pain and also controls excessive blood loss during mensuration.

❖ It has the ability to balance pH levels in the vagina.

❖ It is also useful in male impotency and also decreases the inflammation in the sexual organs.

❖ Due to its cooling effect it is helpful in reducing inflammation in digestive conditions. It is useful in symptoms of hyperacidity because it reduces the secretion of stomach acid and protects the stomach linings.

# CHAPTER 23

## Shankhpushpi- A Memory Booster

One can not acquire a comprehensive knowledge of a particular science unless one studies other sciences too

Susruta

Shankhpushpi – a herb widely used in Ayurvedic medicine as a brain tonic and memory enhancer. Its botanical name is *Convolvulus plunricaulis* is member of *Convulvulaceae family*. Many modern *Ayurvedic* practitioners and authors are of opinion that Shankhpushpi is a gift of nature. It is indicated as a brain tonic and memory booster, digestive, appetite stimulant. Shankhpushpi has been used for centuries as a means to promote higher intelligence and a more expanded world view. The herb has been used in *Ayurveda* for rejuvenating nervous functions. The herb works primarily by supporting the central nervous system. It is a natural tonic for mental development of children. It is also used to treat various disorders related to nervous weakness, problems like insomnia, loss of memory, mental as well as physical fatigue etc.

**Shankhpushpi Herb Information**

**1. Nomenclature**

Family Name*: Convulvulaceae*
Scientific Name*: Convolvulus plunricaulis* Linn
Sanskrit name: Shankhpushpi, Mangalya kasums.
English name: Shankhpushpi
common name: Shankhpushpi

## 2. Bio-energetics

Rasa: Katu, Kashaya
Guna: Guru, Sara, Snigdha, Pichchila
Virya: Ushna
Vipaka: Madhura
Dosha: VPK+
Karma: Medhakrita, Svarakara, Grahabhutadi

## 3. Biomedical Action

Anti-depressant, analgesic, tonic, alexiteric, alternative, astringent.

## Habitat

The plant, shankhpushpi is often found in India and neighboring country Myanmar. The plant can be found in variety of places including sandy and rocky surfaces particularly in North India. In Chhattisgarh, shankhpushpi occurs as wasteland plant. Although for agriculture scientists, it is harmful unwanted weed that compete with agricultural crops for light, moisture and food but for the natives and traditional healers, it is valuable medicinal herb. This plant belongs to *Convulvulaceae* family and usually flowers during September and October.

## Botanical Characters

Shankhapushpi is a perennial herb that seems like morning glory. Its branches are 30- 50 cm long which spread on the ground. Leaves are 2 mm in size, elliptical in shape are located at alternate positions. The flowers are blue in colour, size 5mm. In July, it produces minute, flowers on short, spiky stems, and in September it fruits, producing blackish-purple, globular berries

## Chemical Constituents

Different types of chemical constituents have been reported in shankhpushpi. They are sugars like D-glucose, maltose, rhamnose, sucrose and starch, and certain other bio-chemicals. opoletin, three coumarins, β-sitosterol, tropane alkaloids, kaempferol, convoline, convolidine, convolvine, confoline, convosine, palmitic acid (66.8%), linoleic acid (2.3%), and straight chain hydrocarbon hextriacontane, 20-oxodotriacontanol, tetratriacontanoic acid and 29-oxodotriacontanol. It contains glycosides, coumarins, flavonoids, alkaloids. "Shankha pushpine I"s believed to be the principal active agent responsible for different benefits.

## Plant Part Used

The whole plant is used in Ayurvedic system of medicine.

## Health Benefits

Shankhapushpi has wide spectrum of properties and medically useful benefits

- ❖ Results of the laboratory trial on animals showed that Shankhpushpi extract reduced neurotoxicity of aluminum chloride to a significant extent. The results indicate that shankhapusphi not only effective as a stress reliever and an anti-depressant, but it can also reduce the effect of toxins in the brain.
- ❖ Results of the another laboratory trial showed an improvement in memory after administering with shankhpushpi extracts.
- ❖ Shankhpushpi is having remarkable pain killing or analgesic properties which is very similar to a morphine induced ones. These pain killer properties are very much useful in dealing with rheumatic pains, arthritis, osteoarthritis etc.
- ❖ The thyroid gland is a very important gland which regulate the rate of metabolism. Over production of thyroid hormones is clinically called hyperthyroidism disease which can lead to

uncontrollable weight gain. Hyperthyroidism can be controlled by taking shankhpushpi extracts on a regular basis.

❖ Gastric ulcers are generally caused when the excess of acid (HCl) is produced in the stomach. This happen in cases where the eating habits are irregular or too much spicy food in diet. In such cases, if care is not taken at right time, this extra acid can rupture the stomach lining from the inside causing lesions or ulcers. Studies have shown that Shankhpushpi is a very good herb that can reduce gastric ulcers by healing the lesions faster and also by strengthening the mucus membranes and mucosal cells.

❖ According to *Ayurveda*, Shankhpushpi is bitter, pungent, alternative tonic, brightens intellect, improves complexion, increases appetite, useful in bronchitis, biliousness, epilepsy and teething troubles of infants.

❖ From ancient times in India, people from all walks of life (especially students, teachers and philosophers) always using shankhpushpi as natural brain tonic for rejuvenating nervous functions. It is a natural tonic for mental development of children. The herb enhances brain power such as learning, memory and the ability to recall, intelligence and concentration level. It makes students more receptive to learning and reduces stress of examination and overwork.

❖ Classically, Shankhpushpi was one of the few drugs that were used to reduce stress levels and put the brain in a relaxed state. Studies on animals with induced stress showed that Shankhpushpi possesses stress and depression reducing properties.

❖ Physicaliy, the herb is helpful to eliminate hypertension, anxiety, asthma, stress-related disorders, epilepsy, urinary disorders, constipation, and numerous neurodegenerative diseases including dementia and Alzheimer's disease.

❖ Sankhpushpi is one of the best and prominent natural medicine which helps in improving memory at all ages.

❖ It is also used to treat various disorders related to nervous weakness problems like insomnia, mental as well as physical fatigue etc.

❖ Shankhpushpi is a very wonderful brain tonic that stimulates the brain to improve its ability and capacity.

❖ The whole herb is used medicinally in the form of decoction with cumin and milk in fever, nervous debility, loss of memory, also in syphilis. Decoction was given in cases of malarial fever.

❖ The leaves are made into cigarettes and smoked in chronic bronchitis and asthma.

❖ The plant is useful in internal haemorrhages.

❖ The oil promotes the growth of hair. Is used as a tonic, alterative and febrifuge. It is a sovereign remedy in bowel complaints especially dysentery.

❖ The plant is reported to be a prominent memory improving drug. It is used as a psychostimulant and tranquilizer. It is reported to reduce mental tension. The ethanolic extract of the plant reduces total serum cholesterol, triglycerides, phospholipids and nonesterfied fatty-acid.

❖ It is considered as a Rasayana.

❖ Shankhpushpi controls the production of body's stress hormones like cortisol and adrenaline, thus it has reducing effect on stress and anxiety.

❖ Shankhapusphi herb is also used in the treatment of disorders like hypotension, hypertension etc.

❖ It has soothing action on the nervous system so it is used as a tranquilizer for anxiety neurosis and sleeplessness.

❖ Due to its memory enhancing property, it is useful to treat neurodegenerative diseases like dementia and Alzheimer's disease. The extract of herb helps to decrease the total cholesterol level in the blood with the inclusion of phospholipids, triglycerides, and fatty acids.

❖ The herb is also advantageous in rejuvenation therapy and works as tranquilizer and psycho-stimulant.

❖ The plant can be used to treat constipation due to its laxative properties. The herb Shankhpushpi promotes good sleep and brings relief in mental fatigue. Also, it serves to induce a feeling of peace and calm. It is the best herb that can be used to enhance beauty and to nourish all the layers of skin.

❖ The herb has a refreshing effect on overall health and promotes weight gain.

# CHAPTER 24

## Vidanga: A Herb For Intestinal Worms

"The art of medicine consists of amusing the patient while nature cures the disease"

Voltaire

Vidanga is an Ayurvedic herb(*Embella ribes* burm F*)*, popularly known as Vavding' in *Ayurveda*, is a red-listed species belonging to the family *Myrsinaceae*. In sanskrit, this herb is known as jantanasa. Charak, Sushruta, Vagbhatta all renouned ancient rishis recommended vidanga as a therapeutic in treatment of several diseases. Sushruta has identified it as anthelmintic, alternative tonic herb and recommended to cure for various health disorders. It is a germicidal and bactericidal herb. It is considered one of the best Ayurvedic herbs for eliminating intestinal worms and other parasites. A warming herb used for managing all skin diseases, alleviating thirst, and it has a fruit that looks a lot like black pepper and so is sometimes called false lady pepper. It is anti-estrogenic and, used as oral contraceptive. *E. ribes* is a highly valuable medicinal plant with carminative, antibacterial, antibiotic, hypoglycemic, and antifertility properties. It is considered to be vulnerable due to excessive harvesting, because of its many uses.

**Vidanga Herb Information**

**1. Nomenclature**

Family: *Myrsinaceae*
Scientific Name: *Embelia ribes* Burm F

Sanskrit Name: Janatansa
Common Names: *Vellah,* Baberang, Viranga, Vayuvilanga, Vilal, Kattukodi, Embelia
Other Uncommon Names: Black Pepper, White-flowered Embelia, Janntughna, Kapala, Chitratandula, Krmighna, Vella, Krmihara, Krmiripu, Vayavidanga, Bhabhiranga, Baberang, Vayuvilanga, Vizhalari, Vayuvidangam, Vayuvidangalu, Viranga, Chitratandoola, Vayuvilangam, Vizhal, Vrishanasana, Bayabidanga, Vayabidang.

## 2. Energetics

*Rasa: Kashaya, katu*
Virya: ushna, ruksha, laghu
vipica: Laghu
Doshas: V+, PK -
Karma: dipanapachana, bhedana, krimighna, jvaraghna, mutravirechana, raktaprasadana, kushtaghna, vedanasthapana, sandhaniya, *Kapha*vatahara.

## 3. Biomedical Action

Vedanta fruits are astringent, bitter, anthelmintic, depurative, brain tonic, digestive, carminative, stomachic, diuretic, contraceptive, rejuvenating, alternative stimulant, alexiteric, laxative, anodyne, febrifuge & tonic.

## Habitat

It grows everywhere from the Himalayas to Sri Lanka and Singapore and ranges from India to South China and South to Indonesia, East Africa. This species is reported to be vulnerable in the western ghats of Tamil Nadu and Karnataka states of India and at a lower risk in Kerala state of peninsular India. It is well adapted to many different climates and elevation. *E. ribes* grows in semi-evergreen and deciduous forests at an altitude of 1,500 m (5,000 ft), throughout India. It grows in Jammu and Kashmir, Himachal Pradesh, Uttar Pradsh, Assam, and Maharashtra.

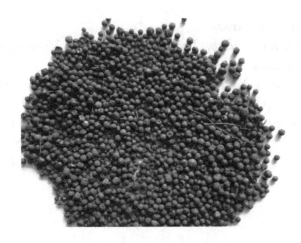

**Vedanga Seeds**

## Botanical Characters

*Vidanga* is a large climbing shrub. The branches are long, slender with long internodes. Leaves are leathery simple, alternate, ellptic-lanceolate, obtusely acuminate, shiny green and glabrous above, silvery below, with scattered, minute sunken glands 6-14 cm long and 2-4 cm broad. Midrib promonant. Stem whitish grey, with a mature girth of 45-72 cms. Flowers are small, white to greensh white, borne in terminal and axillary panicle racemes, the calyx five-lobed, the corolla hairy, with five stamens. The fruit is a smooth globose berry; thin reddish coloured pericarp containing a single seed, found in bunches.

## Chemical Constituents

The most studied chemical in *Vidanga* is embelin (embolic acid), or rather, potassium embelate (2,5-dihydroxy, 3-undecyl-1, 4-benzoquinone). A related quinone found in *Vidanga* is vilangin, a structure of two embelin mocules attached with a $CH_2$ bridge. Other constituents include the alkaloid christembine, a volatile oil, quercitol, tannins and fatty acids.

## Plant Part Used

Fruit, leaves, root, bark

## Health Benefits

Vidanga herb is used both internally and externally. Vidanga has various medicinal benefits which are listed below.

- ❖ Vidanga is used to expel intestinal worms. Powder of vidanga should be taken every morning on an empty stomach. A laxative should be taken in the evening same day. This method is used for destruction of tapeworms, thread worms and round worms.
- ❖ It is bactericidal, hence it is useful in dental carries and toothache. Decoction of this herb is used as a gargle to help prevent dental infections and aches.
- ❖ The herb is considered to be a boon for healthy digestive system. It is used to treat variety of digestive disorders such as flatulence, dyspepsia, loss of appetite, dull abdominal pain and piles. For treatment of chronic constipation, vidanga powder should be mixed with anise seeds powder and should be taken with warm water or buttermilk.
- ❖ The herb is used to treat cold, sinusitis and migraine. To cure cold problem, the fruits should be taken with honey.
- ❖ It is nervine tonic. It is boiled in milk along with garlic is used in disease of the brain and nervous system.
- ❖ This herb is a widely known blood purifier.
- ❖ This herb is diuretic in action. Thus, it is used for treatment of dysuria.
- ❖ A paste prepared from this herb is used for treatment of several skin diseases. It also helps cure skin depigmentation. It is also useful against fever, cough, asthma, cardiac debility, tumour, scabies, psychosis, debility and weakness. The root and bark of *Vidanga* are used similarly to the seed, applied topically as a counter-irritant in joint disease, rheumatism and lung congestion.

❖ The Indian Council of Medical Research in New Delhi reports that *E. ribes* has been found to be safe and effective as a female contraceptive.

❖ Vedanga is one of the best Ayurvedic herbs for supporting the body's natural defenses in the Gastro Intestinal tract. It's hot, pungent and bitter qualities create an environment conducive to digestive health.

❖ Vidanga strengthens the digestive fire and eliminates natural toxins from the GI tract, blood and lymph. Vidanga helps reduce excess *vata* in the colon promoting intestinal comfort. It also regulates the appetite and helps support proper weight.

❖ A paste prepared from this herb is used for treatment of several skin diseases. It also helps cure skin depigmentation.

# CHAPTER 25

## Punarnava: A Powerful Kidney Healing Tonic

---

"Let thy kitchen be thy apothecary; and, let foods be your medicine

Hippocratus

Punarnava is highly valued botanical medicine used since centuries in *Ayurveda*. The word punarnava is a sanskrit word punar means once again /regaining/restoring and 'nava' stands for new. "Punarnava" literally means, one which renews the body or what restores youth. The scientific name (Latin name) of Punarnava is *Boerhavia diffusa* Linn and it belongs to *Nyctaginace*ae family. The plant *B. diffusa* was named in honor of a famous Dutch physician of the 18$^{th}$ c entury. Hermann Boerhaave. Sages of ancient times consumed the roots and leaves of this herb and acquired healh, youthfulness and longivity. In the ancient Ayurvedic texts the Charak Samhita and Sushrita Samhita there is a mention of this plant for the treatment of several diseases. The plant is found as perennial spreading herb in various locations across India. Commonly known as Hog or pig weed and spreading hog weed. It is bitter in taste and has cooling effect. As a bronchodilator and expectorant, it is used in congestive cardiac failure, chronic bronchitis, bronchectasis and plural effusion.

### Punarnava Herb Information

### 1. Nomenclature

Family Name:: *Nyctaginaceae*
Scientific Name: *Boerhaavia diffusa* Linn
Sanskrit Name: Punarnava, Shothagni, Varshabhu

English Name: Punar-nava Hogweed, Horse purslane, Pigweed
Common Name: Moto Satodo, Santhi, Survari

## 2. Bioenergetics

Rasa: Madhura, Tikta, Kasaya
Guna: Laghu
Virya: Ushna
Vipaka: Madhura
Dosha Effect: KV -, P+
Dhatu: Plasma, Blood

## 3. Biomedical Action

Carminative, anti-inflammetory, anti-convulsant, analgesic, diuretic, expectorant, tonic, hepatoprotective, laxative, spasmolytic, antibacterial, analgesic.

## Habitat

Genus *Boerhaavia*, consisting of 40 species is dispersed in tropical and subtropical regions and warm climate of the globe. It is found in Sri lanka, Australia, Sudan and Malay Peninsula, extending to Africa, America, China, and Islands of the Pacific. Among 40 species of Boerhaavia, only six species are found in India, namely *B. diffusa, B. erecta, B. rependa, B. chinensis, B. hirsute* and *B. rubicunda. B. diffusa,* is found in warmer parts of the country and throughout up to 2,000 m altitude in the Himalayan region especially during rainy seasen. It is a perennial, spreading hogweed, commonly occurring abundantly in waste places, ditches and marshy places during rains. The herb occurs naturally in hilly terrain. The herb mostly seen in gravel soil areas which is known as Patharchatta. Generally it is seen on roadside. The plant is also cultivated to some extent in West Bengal. B. diffusa grows throughout India, Bangla Desh, Burma, Sri Lanka and in many tropical countries throughout year but dries during the summer.

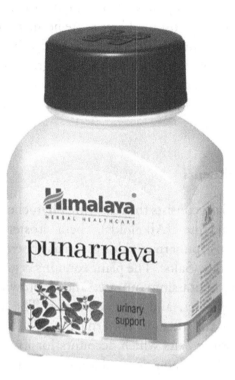

**Punarnava Product**

## Botanical Characters

*Boerhaavia diffusa* is a perennial creeping weed, prostrate or ascending herb, grows to a height of 2 m, having spreading branches. The plant grows profusely in the rainy season, and matures in the months of October-November. Due to its sticky nature, the plant gets stuck on the clothes of human beings and on the legs of animals and birds, which helps in its dispersal from one place to another. The stem is greenish purple, slender, cylindrical, swollen at the nodes; often more than meter long. Roots well developed, fairly long, 0.2 to 1.5 cm in diameter, yellowish brown coloured. The shape of the leaves varies considerably - ovate-oblong, round, or sub cordate at the base and smooth above. Margins of the leaves are smooth, wavy, or undulate. The upper surface of the leaves is green, smooth, and glabrous, whereas it is pinkish white and hairy beneath. Leaves are up to 5.5 X 3.3 cm in area. The seeds germinate before the onset of the monsoon. Flowers are hermaphrodite, pedicellate, and white, pink, or pinkish-red in colour and minute about 1.5 mm long. The fruits are oval in shape having dull green or brownish colour and about the size of caraway bean. It has two varities i.e. white and red variety of punarnava. Only white variety is basially used for medicinal purpose.

## Chemical Constituents

Generally whole plant consists the following phytochemical constituents; they are punarnavine (Alkaloids), beta-sitosterol (phytosterols), liriodendrin (lignans), punarnavoside (rotenoids), boerhavine (Xanthones) and potassium nitrate (Salts). The plant contains crystalline acid known as boerhavic acid, potassium nitrate, and a brown mass consisting of tannis, phlobapnehes, and reducing sugar. The active principle of punarnava herb is the alkaloid punarnavine. The plant contain large quantity of potassium salts which accounts for its diuretic properties. The herb contain 14 amino acids including 7 essential amino acids.

## Plant Parts Used

Whole Plant, Roots

## Health Benefits

In India since ancient time, punarnava is used by indigenous and tribal people for treating different ailments.

❖ The whole plant of *B. diffusa* is a very useful source of the drug. All the plant parts have different therapeutic applications, so to obtain maximum efficacy different plant parts should be used separately. Punarnava is well known anti-spasmodic, diuretic, anti-inflammatory agent. It protects kidney functions particularly nephrons, which are usually demaged by undergoing long term diabetes. This herbal medicine is one of the best Rasayana for the kidney and urinary system. It speeds up the filtration process of kidneys and flushes out the excessive fluids and waste products.

❖ Punarnava supports quality of six out of seven categories of dhatus (tissues) viz; rasa dhatu (plasma), majja dhatu (bone marrow and nerves), rakta dhatu (blood), meda dhatu(fat), mamsa dhatu (muscle) and shukra dhatu (reproductive fluids).

❖ It is very effective in treating a disease called dropsy, a condition wherein excess of watery fluid gets accumulated in the tissues and body cavities. A liquid extract of punarnava stimulates urine secretion and discharge. Thus excess of watery fluid gets removed.

❖ Punarnava is mild and well tolerated medicine. It pacifies all the three doshas. It is stomachic, anti – viral, anti- bacterial myocardial stimulant; herb is useful in anaemia, jaundice, asthma, and an antidote for snake venom.

❖ The aqueous crude extract from the dried roots also found significantly active against a number of viruses – mung bean yellow mosaic virus, bean common mosaic virus.

❖ Roots of plant help killing intestinal worms.

❖ It is an excellent blood tonic with alternative and rejuvenative properties.

❖ Hot bandage of the root is also applied with heartening results in arthritis pain. The seeds are also used in lumbago. In arthritis related disorders, punarvana guggal is highly useful.

❖ Punarnava effectively reduces fever especially malarial fever.

❖ It is very useful medicine for gonorrhea. The roots are used in scanty urine. ascites, anasarca and internal inflammation.

❖ Punarnava can easily remove kidney stone by dissolution.

❖ The root juice is used to cure urinary disorders, leucorrhea, rheumatism, and encephalitis. *B. Diffusa* roots have been widely used for the treatment of dyspepsia, enlargement of spleen.

❖ Punarnava is an excellent blood tonic with alternative and rejuvenative properties. The root of this plant is influential Rasayana for diseases affecting kidneys, heart and lungs. The roots are analgesic, laxative, diuretic, anti-diabetic, anti-convulsant and expectorant. The roots also have hepatoprotective actions. It reduces lung and peripheral oedema, is anti-rheumatic in painful and swollen joints, improves renal function, breaks up renal calculi, and is valuable in nephrotic syndrome.

## Home Remedies

- ❖ In stomach colic, 5 g dose of Punarnava Powder is helpful.
- ❖ Punarnava Powder 1 to 3 g with a glass of milk once or twice a day acts as a good energy tonic.
- ❖ Take 1 tsp "Punarnava Powder" and a pinch of "Sunti (Dry Ginger Powder)" with milk in inflammatory conditions.
- ❖ Apply paste of Punarnava on injured wounds as it is helpful in drying up the oozing wound.
- ❖ For the treatment of urticaria, administere punarnava with dry ginger.
- ❖ The fresh juice of its roots instilled into eyes, mitigates the ailments of the eyes like night blindness and conjunctivitis.
- ❖ The paste applied on the wounds, dries up the oozing. Internally, punarnava is beneficial to treat a wide range of diseases.
- ❖ The alcoholic extract of roots and leaves of plant have powerful inflammatory properties. Oil prepared from the roots mixed with sindhuvara (nirgundi) is applied externally in case of joint pain.

# CHAPTER 26

## Haridra: Nature's Precious Medicine

As a matter of fact, an ordinary desert supports a much greater variety of plants than does either a forest or a prairie.

*Ellsworth Huntington*

*Curcuma longa Linn is* also known as haridra or turmeric belongs to ginger family *Zingiberaceae*. It grows in the tropical regions of India. Haridra affectionately called kitchen queen and is the principal spice of every Indian kitchen. It is a indispensable spice and without turmeric one can not deam of cooking. Haridra is available in market both as powder or as fresh/dry roots. It is also well known for its anti-bacterial activity, anti-inflammatory, analgesic and healing qualities. It has an earthy aromatic and spicy fragrance. Its complexion enhancing property, is used in Indian wedding and in many religious ceremonies in India. Haridra assists in eliminating the undesirable fats from the body; corrects metabolism rate and reduces anaemia, diabetes and liver problems. It has slightly bitter taste. Turmeric is one of the best blood purifier. Haridra has anti-cancerous properties. It is one of the most prestigious and powerful plant on earth and being used as drug by ancient people of India. Haridra when it is in the spice form, it can be very easily identified as it comes with a mesmerizing yellow colour and used in flavouring foods and imparting yellow colour and taste. It is known as indinan saffron. The origin of haridra is not known but it is believed to originate from southern Asia, most probably India. The roots can be eaten raw or ground to a powder after drying. Turmeric is also used as a natural dye and is a part of cosmetics. It has many medicinal properties and is used as a household anti-septic and anti-inflammatory medicine. Turmeric is common home medicine. Without any medical background, people of India know its medicinal value since thousands of years.

## Haridra Herb Information

### 1. Nomenclature

Family Name:: *Zingiberaceae*
Botanical Name: *Curcuma longa* Linn
Sanskrit Name: Haridra, Aushadhi, Gouri, and Kanchan
English Name: Turmeric
Common Name: Turmeric, Curcumin, Haridra, Haldi,

### 2. Bioenergies

Rasa: Tikta, Katu
Guna: Ruksha, Laghu
Virya: Ushna
Vipaka-Katu
Dosa effect: KPV +
Karma: dipanapachana, grahi, jvaraghna, krimiaghna, chedana, raktaprasadana, shothahara, chakshushya, varnya, kushtaghna, saindhaniya, kaphapittahara
Prabhava: Purifies skin and complexion.

### 3. Biomedical Action

Alterative, analgesic, antibacterial, anti-inflammatory, antioxidant, antiseptic, antispasmodic, appetizer, astringent, cardiovascular, carminative, cholagogue, digestive, diuretic, stimulant, and vulnerary.

### Habitat

*Curcuma* grows on forest margins river banks, and in clearings. It can sustain drought condition. In dry season, it loses its leafy parts and survives as underground rhizomes. Thought to be native to eastern India. It is believed that haridra reached China before the 7th century, it was introduced in East Africa in the in 8th century and West Africa in the 13th century. It reached Jamaica in 18th century. Currently, it is widely cultivated across the globe, but large scale commercial production is concentrated in India and South East Asian countries. India aone produce 9 lakh tonnes of turmeric. Some *Curcuma* species also produce tuberous roots, which act as an additional store of food and water. In China, *Curcuma* is mainly produced in the provinces Zhejiang, Sichuan, etc. Turmeric (*Curcuma longa*) and several other species of the *Curcuma* genus grow wild in *the* forests of Southern Asia including India, Indonesia, Indochina, nearby Asian countries, and some Pacific Islands including Hawaii. Haridra is not found in true wild state, although in some constituencies, it appears to have become naturalized. Haridra has been grown in India since ancient time. Curcuma Longa is a tropical plant, and it grows in a humid warm weather with a lot of rainfall. Appropriate temperature for Turmeric is between 20 °C and 30 °C (68 °F and 86 °F). It needs light for growing, then open fields are the best for this plant. In India it is found every where especially it is found in Andhra Pradesh, Tamil Nadu, Orissa, Karnataka, Gujarat Bengal and Maharashtra where there is large area under commercial cultivation.

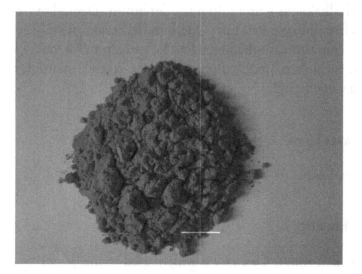

**Haridra Powder**

## Botanical Characters

Haridra is a perennial plant, with a short stem, that attains a height of up to 90 cm long. Roots anout 50 cm long cylindrical with thick sessile tubers, oblong that are intensely orange-yellow when cut or broken. The leaves are simple, quite large in proportion to the stem, the petiole as long as the leaf, oblong-lanceolate, glabrous, entire and acute, 30-45 cm long to 12.5 cm wide. The funnel shaped yellow flowers are borne in spikes, concealed by the sheathing petioles.

## Chemical Constituents

Haridra contributes 2.4 % of pigments called curcuminoids and 3.8 % essential oil containing different sesquiterpenes. Turmeric is fully loaded with hundreds of chemical compounds, each with a distrinct biological activities. they are anti-biotic, cancer preventive, anti-tumor, anti-inflammatory and there are at least 10 different anti-oxidants. The list goes on and on. We can say that turmeric is a complete pharmacy in its own right, with literally hundreds of different chemicals and activities on its shelves.. And amongst all chemicals, there are three chemicals which are the most extensively researched. They are three gold-coloured alkaloidal Curcuminoids: Curcumin, Demethoxy-curcumin, and Bisdemethoxy-curcumin. One hundred gram of edible portion of rhizome contains carbohydrates 69.4%, protein 6.3%, fats 5.1%, fibres it contains calcium, iron and phosphorus, carotene, thiamin, niacin. Its caklorie value is 349.

## Plant Parts Used

Rhizome. Leaves.

## Health Benefits

Since ancient times, *Curcuma* is widely used in medicines.

❖ In the Indian *Ayurveda* system of herbal medicine, haridra is known as strengthening and warming herb for the entire body.

❖ In India, traditionally turmeric is advocated to improve intestinal normal flora, to eliminate intestinal worms, for relief of arthritis and swelling, as a blood purifier, to warm and promote proper metabolism correcting both excesses and deficiencies, to relieve gas, to cleanse and strengthen the liver and gall bladder.

❖ Haridra is an excellent medicine for treating liver disorders, piles, jaundice, loss of appetite, anaemia, constipation.

❖ It is used for various urinary disorders like diabetes, painful urination and enlarged prostate.

❖ It is a traditional medicine against leucorrhoea, menorrhagia, painful menstruation, fistula in anus, enlarged lymph gland, sinus and fever.

❖ It is used to improve digestion, to improve intestinal flora, for soothing action in cough and asthma, as antibacterial and anti-fungus and in any condition of weakness or debility.

❖ Traditionly haridra is used as tonic, a carminative for diarrhoea, for liver problems and jaundice and as cancer remedy.

❖ Scientists have proved that chronic inflammation plays a significant role in development of cancer. Petroleum ether extract and alcohol extracts of haridra exhibited anti-inflammatory activities, which is effetive against cancer cells. This effect is attributed to the presence of essential oil containing ar-turmerone.

❖ A reduction in side effects of chemotherapy and radiation therapy concomitant improvement in quality of life with increase in life-span of cancer patients was observed using *C. longa*.

❖ It balances *vata* and *kapha*. Because of its dryness, pungent and bitter taste, it balances *kapha*. Due to bitterness, it balances *pitta*. Hence it balances all the three doshas.

❖ A formulation of Haridra khanda is widely used in the treatment of allergy and urticaria.

❖ It is used externally and internally in skin diseases caused due to impurities of blood. Haridra raises RBC count and purify impure blood.

❖ Haridra powder is used internally for blood purification, skin blemishes and allergic conditions.

❖ The rhizome of turmeric is stimulant and aromatic.

❖ It is a skin tonic, provides royal lustre and glow, imparts youthful, vitality and vigour.

❖ It is diuretic, wound healer, expectorant, analgesic, germicidal, anti-flatulent, anti-inflammatoty, bone setter, protector of eyes and eye vision.

❖ Externally used in treartment of scabies, itching, boils, eczema, abscesses.

❖ Internally it is used in the treatment of asthma, cough. cold, fever, obstinate skin diseases, urticaruia, jaundice, parasitic infections, constipation.

❖ In one piolet project, adding turmeric to regular exercise provided enhanced cardiovascular fitness in postmenopausal women.

❖ In another study turmeric had improved joint pain and stiffness, physical, social function in arthritis patients.

❖ A piolet study demonstrated improved symptoms and reduced medications from oral turmeric in patients with ulcerative colitis and chrohn's disease.

❖ Turmeric is a potent antioxidant and anti-inflammatory. Results indicates that it can suppress tumor promotion and metastasis and therefore has enormous potential as an anticancer agent.

## Other Uses

❖ Rhizomes are boiled, dried and made into powder, which gives a yellow colour and which is used largely as colouring agent and as condiments entering largely into the composition of Indian pickles and curry powder.

❖ Now a days it is used for beauty care and skin to improve complexion and overall beuty. Haldi is used at the time of marriage for both bride and her groom.

❖ It is often used as food supplement and indespensible ingredient of curry powder.

❖ In Asia, Turmeric is eaten as a food both raw and cooked. While turmeric root resemble with that of ginger root, it is less fibrous and is more chewable, crunchy, and succulent. The fresh root has a somewhat sweet and nutty flavour mixed with its bitter flavour.

As a result, it is pleasant to eat and not difficult to chew. It is sometimes chewed plain or chopped up and part of raw salads.

❖ It is grind in a mortar to make a paste to mix with other spices for flavouring in curries. Currently, the dried root powder as the base of most curries in India and other nearby countries.

## Home Remedies

❖ To expel intestinal worms, mix pinch of salt in 20 ml of raw turmeric taken daily early in the morning for few days.

❖ In painful piles turmeric gives great relief.

❖ In catarrh and coryza, the inhalation of fumes of burning turmeric gives instant relief.

❖ For the control of chronic diarrhoea, turmeric and alum powder in 1:20 proportion is blown into ears.

❖ In the treatment flatulence, dyspepsia, and weak state of stomach, 15 – 20 grains haridra twice day is advised.

❖ A paste of turmeric alone or combined with neem leaves is used in ring worms, eczema, itching, and other parasitic skin diseases.

❖ Smoke generated by sprinkling powder turmeric over burnt charcoal will relieve scorption sting when affected part is exposed to a smoke for few minutes.

❖ Milk boiled with turmeric rhizome and then sw Sprain, inflammatory conditions of joints and burns are the main indications for local application of haridra paste eetened with sugar give instant relief to cold.

❖ Intestinal disorders and chronic diarrhoea are controlled by taking rhizome juice mix with buttermilk.

# CHAPTER 27

## Nagkeshar: A Nervine Tonic

A man doesn't plant a tree for himself. He plants it for posterity.

Alexander Smi

*Mesua ferrea* Linn, generally known as Nagkesar in India. It is a species in the family *Clusiaceae*. It is believed to be native to tropical Sri Lanka but also cultivated in Indochina, Assam, Southern Nepal, and the Malay Peninsula. Nagkeshar is an ornamental tree whose flowers and flower buds are used in folk cosmetics. In Malaysia flowers are used to stuff pillows and cushions. In Sri lanka the tree often cultivated around Buddhist's vihar. The seed oil is used for soap making, lubricating and illuminating, while its fruits are edible. It produces one of the hardest deep dark red timber in the world, because of this unique character, it's wood commonly used for preparing railway sleepers, poles, furnitures etc. Nagkeshar has been described as bitter and pungent in taste and hot, sharp, dry and light in effect. It is a poisonous herb yet because of valuable medical properties it carries importance. It alleviates *kapha* and *vata* but aggravates *pitta*. Dry rhizomes of nagkeshar contain a volatile, yellow aromatic oil. It also has a bitter substance known as acorin.

**Nagkeshar Herb Information**

**1. Nomenclature**

Family Name: *Clusiace*
Scientific Name: *Mesua ferrea* Linn
Sanskrit Name: Nagkeshar

English Name: Mesua, Cobra's saffron
Common Name: Nagesar, Nag kesar, Gansau, Nagesuri, Narmiska, Deyana, Nagechampa.
Synonyms: Nagakeshara, Nagakesara, Nag keshar, Ahipushpa, Kanakahva, Ibha, kanchanahvaya, Nageeya, Kinjilka, Kesahara, Champeya, natam, Nagam, Nagarenuka, Panchabhuvayam, Phanipannagam, Rukmam, Suvarnam, Naga Kinjalka Kanaka, Hemapushpa, Kanchana, Hema Kanchana

## 2. Bioenergies

Rasa: Kashaya, Tikta, katu
Guna: Ruksha, Laghu, teekshna
Virya: Ushna
Vipica: Katu
Dosa effect: KP+
Karma: Deepan, Krimighna, Hridya, Uttejak, Panchan, Vedanasthapan, Uttejak, Vajikaran, Mutrajanan, Kusthaghna, Balya, Durgandhanashana, Svedapanayan, Jvaraghna, Vishagna

## 3. Biomedical Actions

The flowers are astringent, bitter, acrid, mildly heating, anodyne, sudorific, digestive, carminative, constipating, anthelminthic, diuretic, alexipharmic, expectorant, stomachic, haemostatic, aphrodisiac, febrifuge and cardiotonic.

## Habitat

It is distributed in forests of Western ghats from South Kanara to Travancore, evergreen forests of north Kanara to South Konkan. it is also found in mountains of eastern Himalaya and Assam, East Bengal, Burma, Andamans. Common on the eastern Himalayas, east Bengal and Assam, Burma and Andemanns. It is cultivated in gardens.

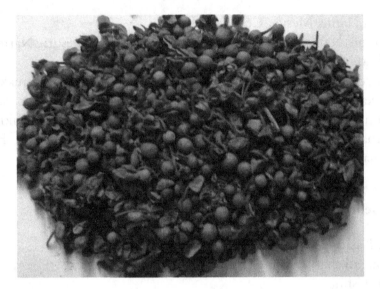

**Nagkeshar Fruits**

## Botanical Characters

Nagkeshar is a medium-sized evergreen tree up to 20 m tall, often buttressed at the base with a trunk up to 1 m. in diameter. Stem bark is, smooth, ash coloured, grey turning to dark brown to reddish. The leaves are alternate, linear, lanceolate, oblong, 5-15 cm long, 3- 5.5 cm wide tapering at both the ends, upper side shining, lowered with a white waxy powder. Flowers are large 4–7.5 cm. solitary or in bunches of two or three, white, yellow or red and fragrant. Fruits ovoid to globose, woody and 2.5 – 5.0 cm. Seeds are 1- 4 shining, dark brown with fleshy and oily cotyledons The wood is extremely hard. It is used for railroad ties and structural timber.

## Chemical Constituents

The flowers of *Mesua ferrea* contain a yellow-coloured highly fragrant essential oil, the stamens specifically containing mesuanic acid, amyrin, sitosterol, and the biflavonoids mesuaferrone A and B. Scientists have also isolated a group of xanthones from *M. ferrea*, including euxanthone, dehydrocycloguanadin, jacareubin, and mesuaxanthones A and B. The seed contains the coumarin mesaugin, the lactones mesuol, mesuone, and mammeisin, as well as a fixed oil comprised of oleic, stearic, palmatic and linoleic acids. Its seeds, kernels forming 53 to 73 % of the weight of the seeds yield in 60-77 % a viscous redish to dark brown oil with a disagreeable odour and bitter taste. Its unripe fruits known to contain resinous oil and the pericarp the tannin. Its flower-stamens, known as kesara contain two bitter substances and a yellow matter.

## Plant Parts Used

Stamens, fruits, flowers, flower buds, seeds, leaves, bark and oil of the plant are used medicinally.

## Health Benefits

Plant material is being used for vide variety of disesases.

- ❖ It is useful in the treatment of acidity of stomach, vomiting, loss of appetite, burning sensations in the chest after taking food, blood vomiting, gastritis, peptic ulcer and pain in intestines.
- ❖ It is also used in the treatment of bronchitis, cough, asthma, headache.
- ❖ Nagkeshar is also effective against diarrhoea, dysentery, sore throat, hicupps, liver disorders, heart diseases, bleeding piles and excessive menstrual bleeding.
- ❖ Externally it is used in the treatment of scabies, eczema and ulcers.
- ❖ Its flower and stamens form a major drug Nagpuspha or Nagkeshar in indigenous system of medicine. This is used as stomachic, expectorant, astringent.
- ❖ They are useful in cough, leprosy, scabies, skin diseases, pruritus, pharyngodynia, vomitting, dysentry, haemorrids, ulcers, burning sensation of feet, depsia, impotency, leucorrhoea, and cardiac debility. The seed oil is used in skin diseases. Pericarp of fruit is astringent and stomachic.
- ❖ Seed oil is analgesic. Saffron is deodrant, antidiaphoretic and stimulant. Hence seed oil is used in inflammatory arthritis for

massage and saffron is used in foul smelling, excessive perspiration and wounds.

❖ Stem bark is used as astringent, in combination with ginger as sudorific. Nagakeshar is applied locally over penis in case of impotency due to its stimulant action

❖ Seed oil is used externally in wound, sore, rheumatism.

❖ Dried flowers are used for thrist, excessive perspiration, indigestion, cough.

❖ Bark and roots in the form of tincture, decoction, infusion are used for gastritis and bronchitis.

❖ Being brain tonic, it is useful in brain debility and hysteria.

❖ Important Ayurvedic preparations are Ashwagandharishta, Chwavanprash, Brahma Rasayana, Shringarabhra rasa, Drakshasava, Dashamoolarishta, Lavanbhaskara Churna, Nagakesarandi.

❖ It is appetizer, mainly digestive, antidipsetic, antiemetic, antihaemorrhoid, astringent and vermicide, hence it is used in anorexia, distaste, dipsia, emesis, worms.

❖ Being cardic tonic and haemostatic, it is used in cardic debility, rakta *pitta* and blood disorders.

❖ It is used as an aphrodisiac and as a haemostatic in menorrhagia.

## Home Remedies

❖ Internally it is generally used in form of a, powder, infusion or decoction. For therapeutical use stamens of flower are very useful. These are cleared of foreign particles and dried in shade before preparing out of it. There after powder remain therapeutically active for thre months. For external use a fine paste is prepared using flowers and buds.

❖ Nagkesar mixed with shatadhouta ghee is applied on burning palms and soles. Leaves are applied on head in severe cold.

# CHAPTER 28

## Musta: A Herb for Obesity

A bodily disease, which we look upon as whole and entire within itself, may, after all, be but a symptom of some ailment in the spiritual past

Nathaniel Hawthorne

*Cyperus rotundus* Linn popularly known as 'Nagarmotha' is a member of family Cyperaceae. The genus name Cyperus is derived from an ancient Greek name Cypeiros; while spacies name rotundus is Latin word for round and refers to the tuber. It is a pestiferous perennial weed arising from underground tubers. Musta is a field weed found through-out India. It is known by nut grass in all the southern states. They form an ingredient in poly herbal formulations like health food Amrita Bindu and Ashokarishta, Shadangapaniya, Gangadhara Churna. Recent studies have also suggested that *musta* is very effective against inflammatory bowel diseases. Its rhizomes are used for washing hair. Oil is obtained from tubers and is used by perfumes as fixative. It acts as an antiperspirant and deodorant. Charak described application of herb in diarrhoea, as an appetite stimulant and for skin infection. For people with *pitta* constitution, musta is one of the best digestive stimulants. and it improves absorption in the small intestine, making it invaluable in the treatment of chronic diarrhoea and malabsorption. The plant is native to Africa, southern and central Europe and southern Asia.

## Musta Herb Information

### 1. Nomenclature

Family Name: *Cyperacae*
Scientific Name: *Cyperus rotundus* Linn
English Name: Nut grass
Sanskrit Name: Musta, Mustaka, Mausta, Maustak, Nagar moth
Common Name: Musta

### 2. Bioenergies

Rasa: Kasaya, katu, tikta
Guna: Laghu, ruksha
Virya: Shita
Vipica: Katu
Dosha effect: PK -, V+ in excess
Dhatus: Plasma, Blood, Muscle, Bone marrow / Nerve

### 3. Biomedical Actions

Carminative, astringent, diuretic, hepatoprotective, analgesic, anti-pyretic, nervine tonic, anti-inflammatory, anti-rheumatic, hypotensive, emmenagoggue, anthelmintic, diaphoretic, hepatic, pungent, antifungal, bitter.

### Habitat

*C. rotundus* is a cosmopolitan weed found in all tropical, subtropical and temperate regions of the world. It is found throughout south India. In India, it is common in open, disturbed habitats to an elevation of about 1800 m. It grows widely on banks of streams and rivers. It is found in all districts throughout India.

## Botanical Characters

Nut grass is a perennial shrub that attains a height of up to 40 cm. It has a dark green thin stem. The leaves are long, flat and sharp, with prominent nerves, several leaves, size, 9-15 x 0.1-0.2 cm. The plant produces rhizomes, tubers, basal bulbs and fibrous roots below ground, and rosettes of leaves, and umbels above the ground. Stems sparsely tufted erect. The branches are long with three edges. The flowers are tiny, total number 10 to 20., flowers pale or purplish. It is also bisexual. Flowers in summer and fruits in winter. It has tuberous roots or rhizomes that are fragrant.

## Chemical Constituents

Scientists have reported 27 different chemical componants from *C. rotundrus*. They are sesquiterpene, hydrocarbons, ketone, monoterpene, epoxides, aliphatic alcohols and some unidentified components. Copadiene and epoxyquaine have also been detected. Using chromatography and spectroscopic techniques, various characteristics of the essential oils have been studied. Cyperine is the major constituent in the plant, which gives nut grass its pharmacological properties

## Plant Parts Used:

Rhizome

## Health Benefits:

Principal health benefits of musta includes

❖ *C. rotundrus* is recommended for intestinal problems, indigestion, fever, vomiting intestinal cramps, irritable bowels, dysentery, diarrhoea, flatulence, sluggish lever, dysmenorrhea, cold, flu and congestion.

❖ The herb is extremely helpful in cases of menopause, menstrual cramps, irregular menstruation and blockage there in.

- ❖ Musta is used for obesity.
- ❖ Musta is a tonic for liver and heart, a drug for the hypertension.
- ❖ Alcoholic/aqueous extract of rhizome displayed analgesic, antipyretic, diuretic and hypotensive activities which is attributed to triterpenoid.
- ❖ Working of spleen, liver and pancreas get synchronized by herb.
- ❖ It is beneficial in bloody stool, urine and vomiting blood, colic, convulsions, moodiness and depression.
- ❖ Musta rhizome increases appetite, lowers blood pressure, reduces breast tumour.
- ❖ Traditionally musta has been used in chronic diarrhoea. It is found useful in patients having diarrhoea with mucus. It is commonly prescribed as antiperspirant and deodorant in case of patients with fever.
- ❖ The oil was found to be effective against various bacterial and fungal species viz. *Bacillus subtilis, Escherichia coli, Pseudomonas aeruginosa and Staphylococcus aureus, Candida parapsilosis, Aspergillus flavus, Aspergillus fumigatus* and *Fusarium oxysporum* in different concentrations
- ❖ It cures *kapha* and *pitta* disorders, dyspepsia, indigestion, dysuria, poisonous affections.
- ❖ The drug is also useful in loss of memory, epilepsy, and general debility. The paste is applied in skin diseases and eye disease.
- ❖ It is observed that oral administration of drug produces significant reduction in body weight and that it lowers blood pressure hypertensive obese patients.
- ❖ Recent studies revealed that the biologically active constituents of the extract facilitate the free circulation of blood by removing congestion and improving the quality of blood.
- ❖ This herb is sometimes used for intestinal disorders such related conditions. liver, menstrual disorder, relieves menstrual pains, digestive stimulant, memory and nervine tonic.
- ❖ It is concluded that *C. rotundrus* rhzome extract, probably through its antioxidant properties could have exerted a potent antiepileptic effect

❖ It is a common weed which is represented by several types growing in India. Musta plant's blackish rhizome is slightly fragrant and essential oil of rhizome is used as perfume and to repel insects.

## Other Uses

❖ The results of one trial suggested that the essential oils of these *Cyperus* species can serve as a potential source of natural mosquitocidal agents.

❖ A study was conducted to test the phytochemical screening and insecticidal testing of *C. rotundrus*. It is more effective than Carbamate and has almost the same efficacy as that of organophosphate.

❖ Result obtained from the laboratory experiment showed that the tuber extracts are more effective for repellency of the entire mosquito vector even at a low dose.

## Home Remedies

❖ Decoction of rhizome with stem bits of guduchi and dried ginger is given to treat malarial fever.

❖ Rhizome juice is given in the dose of 25 ml thrice daily for 3 days to treat constipation.

❖ The rhizomes are scraped and pounded with green ginger mixed with honey prescribed in dysentery, gastric and intestinal troubles

❖ Pound one handful of rhizome with mortar and pestle. Prepare decoction or mix pulp with honey. You can use ginger as conjugant.

❖ Fresh tubers are applied to the breast as a galactagogue.

# CHAPTER 29

## Twak: A Remedy For Stomach Ulcer

Doctors give drugs of which they know little, into bodies, of which they know less, for diseases of which they know nothing at all.

Voltaire

Twak popularly known as Cinnmon belongs to the genus Cinnamomum. It is a small tree originating from Sri Lanka. The scientific name is *Cinnamomum zeylanicum* Blume, while in Sanskrit it known as Twak. True Cinnamon is native to Sri Lanka, the southeastern coast of India, while its closely related tree Cassia is native to China. Cinnamon and Cassia are both small tropical evergreen trees with aromatic bark and leaves. Cinnamon is the hardiest among the tree spices, tolerating a wide range of soil types and climatic conditions. The soil conditions are very important, as waterlogged soil will produce a inferior quality of r cinnamon bark. Scientifically ceylon cinnamon (*Cinnamomum zeylanicum Blume*) is only true cinnamon. Although Cassia is also sold as cinnamon being similar to Ceylon cinnamon. Many people love the distinctive flavour and unique aroma of cinnamon. Among all known spices, cinnamon has the highest antioxidant levels. Often cinnamon popularly known as a natural powerhouse of antioxidants, anti-inflammatory, and blood sugar-lowering abilities. For instance, cinnamon taken from the inner bark of tropical trees is also a powerful antioxidant. Cinnamon is rich in natural compounds known as polyphenols. These compounds act like insulin within the body and can help regulate blood sugar levels as well as contribute to healthy blood circulation and heart function.

# Twak Herb Information

## 1. Nomenclature

Family Name: *Lauracaeae*
Scientific Name: *Cinnamomum zeylanicum* Blume
Sanskrit Name: Twak
English Name: Cinnamon, Ceylon Cinnamon
Common Name: Saigon cinnamon, Ceylon cinnamon, Dalcini, Gui, Twak, Yueh-kuei

## 2. Bioenergies

Rasa: Pungent
Guna: Light, dry, penetrating
Dosha effect: V-, P-

## 3. Biomedical Action

Alterative, analgesic, anodyne, anti-bacterial, anti-fungal, anti-infective, anti-oxidant, anti-parasitic, anti-septic, astringent, carminative, diaphoretic, emmenagogue, haemostatic, hypotensive, sedative, stimulates and then depresses the nervous system, stomachic.

## Habitat

The tree grows abundantly in Malabar, Cochin-China, Sumatra, Eastern Islands, Brazil, Mauritius, India and Jamaica. It is cultivated in South India for its aromatic bark. It is also found to a limited extent in eastern India The optimum climate has an average temperature between 27-30°C and 2000- 2500mm of rainfall. The plant grows best in tropical forest with an altitude of 500 m (1,500 ft), wild populations of the plant originally grew only in India and Sri Lanka, however, the cinnamon is now grown in many other areas of the world with similar climates. For examples, the West Indies and the Philippines now have extensive areas under cultivation.

## Botanical Characters

Twak is a small to medium, straight, tropical evergreen tree that grows up to 6 to 12 m. Branches only at the top of the tree. Cinnamon is a beautiful ornamental tree with golden red aromatic bark, dried bark is used as spice. Leaves oblong, alternate, thick, aromatic, dark, shining green with a length of 7 – 18 cm., grow in clusters at the top of the branches. Flowers are small, white, grow in panicles, seldom open and have distinct odour. The tree bears purple berries. New foliage is deep red. The fruit is an oblong berry containing four kidney-shaped seeds, and turns from green to blue and then to a glossy black. Cinnamon has a fragrant perfume and a sweet and aromatic taste.

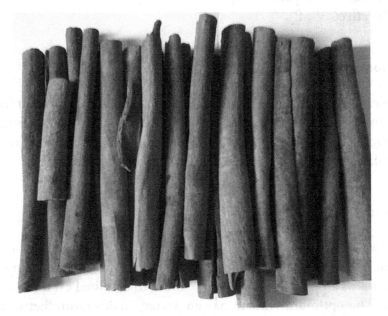

**Twak Bark**

## Chemical Constituents

It contains a significant amount of a mucilaginous substance, which consists mainly of a water extractable L-arabino-D-xylan and an alkali-extractable D-glucan. The bark also contains the diterpenes, cinnzeylanin and cinnzeylanol besides tannins. Cinnamon contain up to 4% oil of cinnamaldehyde, The oil has a pungent, aromatic taste, and contains eugenol, cineol, and terpenes, and trans-cinnamic acid, It also contains phenolic compounds, tannins, catechins, calcium, iron, mucilage, resin, natural sugars, and traces of coumarin.

## Plant Part Used

Bark (bark, or quills, in whole, cut or powdered form)

## Health Benefits

Cinnamon could be described as a natural powerhouse that is filled with anti-inflammatory, anti-oxidants, and blood sugar-lowering abilities.

❖ Recent studies have shown that cinnamon highly effective for 'metabolic syndrome' a 'pre' stage of insulin resistant type 2 diabetes. In Type II diabetes, the pancreas produces insulin, but the body can't use it efficiently to break down blood sugar. Two teaspoons of the cinnamon spice have shown a remarkable effect in people who were not on insulin medication. Cinnamon helps people with diabetes metabolize sugar better.

❖ Twak is recommended in, flatulent dyspepsia, dyspepsia with nausea and intestinal colic. It is known to relieve nausea and vomiting, and because of its mild astringency, it is particularly used for diarrhoea in children.

❖ A study of Indian medicinal plants revealed that may cinnamon potensively be active against HIV.

❖ Cinnamon is a carminative, an agent that helps break up intestinal gas that has traditionally been used to control diarrhoea and morning sickness relieves mild abdominal discomfort caused by excess gas.

❖ Results of the one study showed that Cinnamon "suppresses completely" the cause of most urinary-tract infections caused by *Escherichia coli* bacteria and the fungus *Candida albus* responsible for vaginal yeast infections.

❖ Cinnamon contains the anti-oxidant glutathione and a type of flavonoid. It is believed that cinnamon makes fat cells much more responsive to insulin, the hormone that regulates sugar metabolism and thus controls the level of glucose in the blood.

❖ Cinnamon contains compounds called catechins, which help relieve nausea. The volatile oil in cinnamon bark may also help the body to process food by breaking down fats during digestion.

❖ It stimulates the urinary tract and can be used for problems of the kidneys, edema and urinary retention.

❖ It is a treatment of choice for cough and congestion of the respiratory system. In latest research cinnamon found to reverse the biomechanical, cellular and anatomical changes that occur in the brains of mice with Parkinson's disease.

❖ In Ayurvedic medicine Cinnamon oil is used in external applications for rheumatism, aching joints and stiffness.

❖ It is also used for toothache and sore gums, much like clove oil.

❖ The essential oil component of cinnamon has anti-coagulant properties, which helps to thin blood and improves circulation.

❖ In both India and Europe, cinnamon has been traditionally taken as a warming herb for "cold" conditions, often in combination with ginger *(Zingiber officinale)*. The herb stimulates the circulation, especially to the fingers and toes and has been used for arthritis. Cinnamon is also a traditional remedy for aching muscles and other symptoms of viral conditions such as colds and flu.

❖ It is a drug of choice in abdominal pain, arthritis, asthma, backaches, bloating, bronchitis, candida, cholera, cold or flu with chilliness, aching, sweating but cold skin, constipation, coronary problems, diarrhoea, digestive irritation, dysmenorrhea, excessive menstruation, fevers, flatulence, gastric disorders, haemorrhoids, hypertension, indigestion, nausea, nephritis, parasites, passive gastric/pulmonary/intestinal/renal bleeding, psoriasis, stomach upset, vomiting

❖ The simple touch of cinnamon infuses warmth and energy throughout your body. As part of tea blends, cinnamon improves the taste of less tasty herbs and adds powerful antibacterial power to cold and flu remedies. Cinnamon essential oil is a reliable remedy for athletes foot. It should be diluted with a carrier oil before application. The spice has the ability to stop medication-resistant yeast infections.

❖ It reduces the proliferation of leukemia and lymphoma cancer cells.

❖ Cinnamon has an anti-clotting effect on blood.

## Other Uses

❖ Cinnamon is widely used as a flavouring agent for candy, toothpaste, mouthwashes, and bath and body products. In herbal teas, cinnamon improves the flavour of less palatable herbs. And, of course, it is a staple for baking and cooking. Since it is delicate in flavour, cinnamon is used in dessert dishes.

❖ The spice is used in Indian curries and forms a part of the garam masala.

❖ Both Indian and Sri Lankan cooking Cinnamon is used as a common spice, not only for sweets, but also as an integral part of the well-known spice mixture known as 'curry powder'. It is frequently mixed with honey and taken as tea.

❖ It also exhibits anti-microbial and anti-fungal properties. The anti-microbial action helps to preserve food and can be used in place of common food preservatives. It not only helps to prevent food spoilage by common bacteria, but also by yeasts. Cinnamon is one of the few herbs that can used to treat fungal growths like candida.

## Home Remedies

❖ Chewing and swallowing a small pinch of powdered cinnamon is helpful in treating cough accompanied by spitting of whitish phlegm. The remedy is also helpful to people having cold feet and hands a Smelling cinnamon boosts cognitive function and memory.

❖ People suffering from arthritis should be given half a teaspoon of cinnamon powder, mixed with one tablespoon of honey every morning, before breakfast. It relieves the pain and the patient becomes capable of walking without pain within one month.

❖ Consuming half teaspoon of the cinnamon powder each day helps in reducing blood sugar, cholesterol and triglyceride levels by as much as 20%.

## Caution

❖ Cinnamon should not be consumed by women who are still breastfeeding their child.

❖ The spice is known to cause unwanted effects in sensitive individuals.

❖ It can prove to be toxic, if taken in large doses.

# CHAPTER 30

## Yashtimadhu: A Potent Medicinal Herb

"If people let the government decide what foods they eat and what medicines they take, their bodies will soon be in as sorry a state as are the souls who live under tyranny."-

Thomas Jefferson

*Glycyrrhiza glabra Linn* is scientific name of very popular herb called licorice. Licorice roots carry the sanskrit name of "Yashtimadhu". Yashti means stalk and madhu means sweet. Yashtimadhu is one of the ingredient of 1250 Ayurvedic products in ancient *Ayurveda*. The genus name *Glycyrrhiza* is derived from the Greek term glykos (meaning sweet) and rhiza (meaning root)". The species name glabra is derived from the Latin glaber, which means "smooth" or "bald" and refers to the smooth husks. *Glycyrrhiza glabra* Linn, commonly known as 'liquorice' and 'sweet wood' belongs to *Leguminosae* family. Licorice has a long history of medicinal use in both Eastern and Western systems of medicine. Today, licorice is used as a folk or traditional remedy for stomach ulcers, bronchitis, and sore throat, as well as infections caused by viruses, such as hepatitis. Licorice is one of the principal drugs in Sushruta Samhita. Licorice flavour is found in a wide variety of licorice candies. Licorice has also been used as a medicinal agent in a number of civilizations, dating back to ancient Egypt and China. Medicinal uses have included cough suppression, gastric ulcer treatment, treatment of early Addison disease, treatment of liver disease, and as a laxative. The use of licorice preparations in the treatment of bronchial infections and throat is documented for more than 4,000 years. Next to ginger, licorice is the world's most widely used herbal remedy.

## Yashtimadhu Herb Information.

### 1. Nomenclature

Family name: *Leguminosae*
Botanical Name: *Glycyrrhiza glabra* Linn
Sanskrit Name: Yashtimadhu
English Name: Licorice, Sweet Wood
Common Name: Licorice, Spanish licorice, Russian licorice, Glycyrrhizae radix

### 2. Bioenergies

Rasa: Madhur
Guna: Guru, Snigdha
Virya: Shita
Vipica: Madhur
Dosha effect: KV +
Srotas: Reproductive,
Karma: Yashtimadhu alleviates *vata* and *pitta* dosha

### 3. Biomedical Action

Tonic, expectorant, diuretic, anti-inflamatory, anti-virus, anti-ulcer, anti-biotic, memory stimulator, anti-tussive, anti-arthritic, anti-oxidant, estrogenic.

### Habitat

Licorice is a native of Europe and Asia. It is also found growing in the Australia and America. It tends to grow best in sunny and dry climate. The crop requires relatively low rainfall of around 500mm -700mm., however licorice plant grow in areas receiving average rainfall between 400 to 1200 mm. The crop requires optimum pH between 5.5 to 8.0. There are varieties of licorice with varying appearances viz; Russian,

Chinese, Spanish and Persian. It grows wild but also cultivated in subtropical and warm regions in many parts of the world including India. It is distributed in Southern Europe, Syria, Iran, Afghanistan, Russia, China, akistan and Northern India. This plant is cultivated in Russia, UK, USA, Italy, France, Germany, Spain and China, it is culyivated in Northern India in Punjab and Sub-Himalayan tracts. Large scale commercial cultivation is seen in Spain and England.

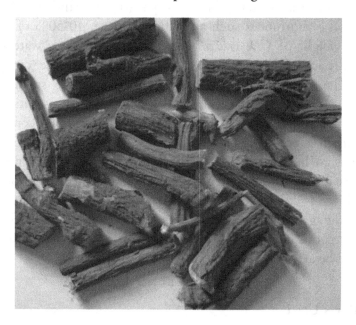

**Yastimadhu Root**

## Botanical Characters

Licorice is a perennial, robust, herbaceous plant growing up to 1.5 m high with an extensive root system consisting of a tap root, root branches, and long runners. The flower petal are blue to purple, white. The leaves are compound, alternate. There is one leaf per node along the stem. The edge of the leaf blade is entire. The woody stalk bears a loose foliage with unpaired pinnate, narrowly lanceolate leaves covered with sticky glandular hairs. The fruit is dry but does not split open when ripe

## Chemical Constituents

The chemistry of licorice root is complex. From the licorice roots a large number of chemical components have been isolated. The principal chemical constituent of liquorice is glycyrrhizin, which is present in the drug in the form of the potassium and calcium salts of glycyrrhizic acid constitute 10 to 25 % of licorice root extract. It is a saponin compound which is 50 times sweeter than cane sugar (sucrose) and encourages the production of hormones such as hydrocortisone. 40-50% of total dry material weight of *Glycyrrhiza glabra* is accounted by water-soluble, biologically active complex. Apart from starch (30%), other components include flavonoids, polysaccharides, pectins, simple sugars, gums, mucilage, tannins, sterols, resin, amino acids, saponin, essential oil, fat, estrogen, glycosides, volatile oil and various other complex components. Glycyrrhizin is considered to be the most common of the Asiatic folk medicines to be used as an anti-inflammatory agent on neutrophil functions including ROS (reactive oxygen species) generation. Thus, Glycyrrhizin is considered as quenching agent of free radicals and also as blocking agent of lipid peroxidation chain reactions. The flavonoids are also responsible for the yellow colour of the root as well as for the health of the arteries

## Plant Parts Used

Roots and rhizomes

## Health Benefits

Licorice is an effective medicine in *Ayurveda* against number of diseases.

❖ The presence of flavonoids confers powerful antioxidant property to licorice. Antioxidant activity of licorice flavonoids was found to be 100 times stronger than that of vitamin E. Currently flavonoids of licorice are strongest antioxidants known.

❖ Glycyrrhzin because of presence of antioxidants neutralize presence of free radicals which stimulate inflammation and swelling of the bronchial passageways in asthma. Licorice increases secretion of mucus in windpipe, which relieves dry cough. once inflammation is removed, windpipe opens up. Patient wil feel ease.

❖ It is proved that licorice extract exhibits anti-viral activity against Varicell zoster, Japanese encephalitis and influenza virus. Because licorice roots can protect the body against number of cancer causing viruses, it has been previously employed in the treatment of HIV.

❖ Licorice was found effective against digestive disorders- peptic ulcers, ulcerative colitis, Crohna disease, chronic gastritis, heartburn, constipation.

❖ Liquorice root (Glycyrrhiza) extract promotes the healing of ulcers of the stomach and mouth. The fact was known for over 2,000 years. It is reported that glycyrrhetinic acid in liquorice extract gives anti-inflammatory effect similar to glucocorticoids and mineralocorticoids

❖ Licorice found to give relief in different immune infections including respiratory infections, urinary tract infection, hepatitis, allergies, herpes, autoimmune disorders etc.

❖ The presence of Glycyrrhizic acid in licorice root can help with nervousness and depression by encouraging the function of the adrenal glands.

❖ The roots of licorice has antispasmodic and estrogenic action which might help in symptoms of menstrual cramps, nasusea, bloating, mood swings.

❖ The extract of liquorice is reported to be an effective pigment lightening agent. It is the safest pigment-lightening agent known with least side effects.

❖ Licorice is effective in the improvement of neuropharmacological activity i.e. intelligence, memory in adolescents.

❖ Because of the presence of saponins, alkaloids and flavonoids, root extract of *Glycyrrhiza glabra,* exhibits potent antibacterial activity. Studies have proved that aqueous and ethanolic extracts of liquorice show inhibitory activity on cultures of *Staphylococcus aureus* and *Streptococcus pyogenes.*

❖ Licorice extract is responsible for its powerful antioxidant activity by means of significant free radical scavenging, hydrogen-donating, metal ion chelating, anti-lipid peroxidative and reducing abilities. Liquorice flavonoids have exceptionally strong antioxidant activity. Antioxidant activity of liquorice flavonoids was found to be over 100 times stronger than that of antioxidant activity of vitamin E.

## Other Uses

❖ Licorice is also found in some soft drinks (eg. root beer) and is in some herbal teas where it provides a sweet after taste.

## Home Remedy

❖ Scientists have demonstrated that individuals who took regular three grams of licorice root extract two times a day for two months had significant reduction in body fat mass.

# PART III
# CLASSICAL RASAYANA

# CHAPTER 31

## Brahma Rasayana: An Antiaging Nervine Tonic

**The oneness of mind and body holds the secret of illness and health.**

Arnold Hutschnecker

*Ayurveda* has given number of herbal products for natural rejuvenation and longivity. Among all, brahma Rasayana is believed to be on top of the list. It is believed that this herbal recipe has been prescribed by Lord Brahma, hence it is called Brahma Rasayana. As per the Ayurvedic texts the famous Rishies of Vaikhanas and Balkhilya group used this brahma Rasayana and acquired youth replacing physique endowed with great memory, intellect, concentration and physical strength and attained immeasurable life span. In spite of its superiority, this formulation is not as popular and widely used as chyawanprash. Brahma rasayana is an herbal jam preparation (similar to chyawanprash); both are amalaki based. The difference between two is chyawanprash is a well-known anti-aging Ayurvedic product with immense effect on respiratory health, mental health and immunity and considered general all purpose rasayana, while brahma Rasayana is another anti-aging Ayurvedic formulation with immense effect on mental health and immunity and considered special purpose Rasayana. It is extremely useful to those who do intensive mental work. Combination of immunity enhancing and antioxidant herbs blended in Brahma Rasayana make, it a very special powerful preparation.

## Composition

It is a herbal preparation containing more than 40 different herbs, and the main ingredients are amalaki fruit (*Emblica officinalis*), haritaki (*Terminalia chebula)* which constitute about 20% and 6.7%, respectively. Important ingredients with their functions are summarized in Table 31.1

### Table 31.1 Composition of Brahma Rasayana

| SR. No. | Name of Herb | Scientific Name | Functions |
|---|---|---|---|
| 1. | Amalaki | *Emblica officinalis* | Acts as Rasayana and is one of the best anti-oxidants known. While providing anti-aging effect, it also improves the functioning of sensory organs. |
| 2. | Haritaki | *Terminalia chebula* | A Rasayana for the mind and nervous system. Through its sharp quality, haritaki strengthens the nervous system, bringing sharpness and clarity to mind, and acts as a carrier for the numerous phytochemicals provided by the other herbal ingredients of this formula. Its sharp quality helps removing mental fog caused by excess *kapha*. Haritaki brings about vitality to the mind through its capacity to penetrate and spread through the nervous system. |
| 3. | Dashamula | Roots of 10 herbs. | Dashmula is a special combination of 10 roots, selected specially for their grounding effect and capacity to balance *vata* dosha, which governs the functioning of the nervous system. |
| 4. | Shankhapushpi and vacha | *Convolvulus pleuricaulis), Acorus calamus* | Excellent memory enhancer, improves speaking capability. Shankapushpi is a calming brain tonic and balances the three doshas. |

| 5. | Pippali | *Piper longum* | A brain tonic strengthening the tejas, mental fire and it brings about clarity and mental strength, removing the weakness of brain, and it heals *vata* related mental disorders. |
|---|---|---|---|
| 6. | Cinnamon | *Cinnamomum zeylanicum* | Remove neural debilities and is a very good appetizer and digestive, while bringing its pleasing warm aroma to this formulation. |
| 7. | Haridra | *Curcoma longa* | Haridra reduces exess *Kapha* and calms the nervous system through its mildly analgesic properties. Haridra – highly recommended anti allergic agent. Good for skin, lungs and fights against cancer. |
| 8. | Cardamom | *Elettaria cardamomum* | Cardamom removes weakness by strengthening mental stamina through increasing agni, the digestive fire. It also contributes to the taste of this formula, providing sense of freshness. |
| 9. | Guduchi | *Tinospora cordifolia* | An immunomodulator is one of the most important divine herb of *Ayurveda*, as it has the capacity to balance all bodily tissues as well as to build up ojas. |
| 10. | Ushir | *Vetiveria zizanoides* | Gives strength to the nerves and brain, provides healing in brain disorders, as well as by reducing excess space element from the brain, helping the individual not to feel "spaced out", and be more grounded. |
| 11. | Mabdukpabi | *Centella asiatica* | Best and most respected Medhya rasayana (mental tonic) herbs, is an excellent memory enhancer, helps to prevent brain weakness and cure mental disorders. |

| 12. | Musta | *Cypendus rotundus* | Excellent brain and nervine tonic, and helps to prevent mental disorders and convulsions. |
|-----|-------|---------------------|------|
| 13. | Bala | *Sida codifolia* | Overall strength |
| 14. | Vidanga | *Embelia ribes* | Vidanga, again considered as one of the best Rasayana, is very good nervine tonic. It fights against toxins and microorganisms bacteria. |
| 15. | Jatiphal | *Myristica fragrans* | Its aromatic qualities gives depth to the taste of this formula while acting as a tonic for mental disorders, preventing convulsions, while being also a good *vata* Shatavari – good for male and female reproductory systems. |
| 16. | Shatwari | *Asparagus racemosus* | Shatavari – good for male and female reproductory systems and for gastric pacifier. |
| 17. | Nagakesar | *Mesua ferrea* | Brain tonic and helping in brain debility. It also prevents as well as heals from schizophrenia. |
| 18. | Bimbi | *Coccinea indica* | Fights against fever. |
| 19 | Jivanti | *Leptadaenia raticulata* | A rejuvenator, cooling, eye tonic. |
| 20 | Licorice | *Glycyrrhiza glabra* | Today, licorice is used as a folk or traditional remedy for stomach ulcers, bronchitis, and sore throat, as well as infections caused by viruses, such as hepatitis. |
| 21 | Punarnawa | *Boerhaavia diffusa* | Cardiotonic, diuretic, helps in anaemic. |
| 22 | Shali rice | *Oriza sativa* | Complete & essential food as it is rich in vitamins, micro nutrients, amino acids & essential elements. |

| 23. | Kans | *Saccharum spontaneum* | Useful in treatment of dyspepsia, burning sensation, piles, sexual weakness, gynecological troubles, respiratory troubles etc |
|-----|------|------------------------|----------------------------------------|
| 24. | Plava (Night Jasmine) | *Nyctanthes arbor-tristis* | In the treatment od piles, dry cough, intestinal worms in children. |
| 25. | Patala Trumpet (root) | *Stereospermum suaveolens* | Powerful Analgesic and Anti inflammatory herb, good cardiac tonic and used in heart diseases. |
| 26. | Bilwa | *Aegle marmelos* | A treatment for diarrhoea. |
| 27. | Shyonaka | *Oroxylum indicum* | Treatment of cancer |
| 28. | Shara | *Serratophyllum submersom* | Enlivening, anti aging group of herb |
| 29. | Gambhari – Coomb Teak (root) | *Gmelina arboera* | It is used in the treatment of all types of *Vata* disorders involving emaciation, lack of strength, pain, stiffness etc. |
| 30. | Rishabhaka | *Manilkara hexandra* | Used in Ayurvedic post natal care of mother and in gynaecological diseases. It is also effective against *Vata* diseases, low back ache It is a good uterine tonic. |
| 31. | Agnimantha | *Premna corymbosa* | Useful in neuralgia, arthritis, muscular dystrophy – useful in premature ejaculation |
| 32. | Prishniparni | *Uraria picta* | Used in depression and psychiatric condition |
| 33. | Brihati | *Solanum indicum* | Analgesic, Respiratory problems · Anti-pyretic · Urinary tract infection |
| 34. | Kantakari | *Solanum xanthcarpum* | Kantkari is useful in treating worms, cold, hoarseness of voice, fever, dysuria, enlargement of the liver, muscular pain, spleen and stone in the urinary bladder. |

| 35. | Sugarcane | *Saccharum officinarum* | Principally used to reduce elevated blood cholesterol levels, aiding in the prevention of cardiovascular disease. It has been shown in many therapeutic trials to be an effective and safe cholesterol-lowering supplement, capable of reducing cholesterol equally as well as most statin drugs used for this purpose. |
| 36. | Jivaka | *Malaxis acuminata* | It is helpful in the smooth functioning of circulatory, nervous system. |
| 37. | Meda | *Litsea monopetala* | |

## Health Benefits

Sages (Rishi) have taken this unique recipe and attained immense longevity, their body were free from ageing effects and became young and energetic, and they were free from diseases and fear, and were endowed with intellect, memory and strength.

❖ Since this brahma Rasayana is prescribed by lord Brahma, it has spiritual value. Person who desires youthful and longevity should consume it. So when one regularly take it, he/she becomes free from diseases and gains longevity and vigour. It increases memory power, mental awareness, calmness, focus, concentration and helps to improve intellect. By providing calmness and serenity, it works wonders in many cognitive and psychological problems, such as memory loss, anxiety and depression.

❖ It restores youthfulness and improves complexion, memory power, will power, body strength, luster, sweetness of voice; increase physical strength and immunity, cures drowsiness, laziness and weakness.

❖ It is a powerful *Ayurvedic* Rasayana, rejuvenating tonic for the brain, mental functions and the nervous system. It also improves mental concentrataion, alertness.

❖ It maintains correct balance of tridoshas. It pacifies the *vata, pitta* and *kapha*, thereby maintains balance of tridosha.

❖ It is supposed to nourish various organs of the body, blood, lymph, flesh, adipose tissue and semen, and thus prevent freedom from chronic degenerative disorders like arthritis and disease of senility.

❖ Brahma Rasayana improves metabolic processes which results in best possible biotransformation and produce the best quality bodily tissue and delay senility and prevent occurrance of other diseases of old age.

❖ Rasayana builds natural resistance against infection.

❖ It invigorates the body in general by sustaining the required balance between anabolism and catabolism.

❖ The ingredients incororporated in Brahma Rasayana are powerful antioxidants which protect the body from aging.

❖ It is said that the herbal preparation provides great strength providing a life span of one thousand years. In ancient times, sages use to enjoy such a long life in healthy disease free state. It is also claimed to be effective in promoting intellect and sense organs. Perhaps this may not be possible in pesent era, but certainly with consumption of brahma Rasayana, one can attain a long disease free life.

❖ It rejuvenates the body and fights against tiredness, fatigue, early grey hairs, wrinkling (skin rejuvenation and hair rejuvenation). It is the best anti aging formula. It also improves intelligence, memory and immune power.

❖ Brahma Rasayana renders it a potential therapy for the prevention of cancer. It is antitumor, minimum side effects of chemotherapy and radiation, possible treatment of cancer. Rasayana therapy fight against denerative changes occurring in the body and for mainteaining health through out life span of the individual.

❖ It also improves intelligence, memory and immune power. It is a good natural rejuvenating anti-aging formula. The person who take brahma Rasayana regularly, his body becomes compact like steel.

❖ This is a fantastic and truly unique but very well balanced formula having combination of herbs for the mind, body, brain and nervous system. This ancient formula of Brahma Raasayana has earned its praise and reverence as one of the most astonishing examples of the deep knowledge of the ancient Rishis of India for the benefit of human kind.

❖ It provides excellent year round protection, gently detoxifies and promotes healthy cellular regeneration throughout the body.

# CHAPTER 32

## Chyawanprash: Ageless Wonder

The treatments themselves do not cure the condition. They simply restore the body's healing abilities"

Leon Chaitow, N.D., D.O

Chyawanprash is most respected, time tasted anti-aging tonic which is used in India with same enthusiasm for the past 4,000 years. For centuries, it has been used to promote youth, vigour, vitality and longivity. Although chyawanprash is a complex mixture of more than 40 ingredients, it is considered as a single unit in *Ayurveda*. It helps to maintain youthfulness by *renewing* tissues and counterattacking degeneration process in the body. Chyawanprash is considered as an excellent tonic for aged persons as well as children. There are numerous stories and legends about the discovery and first use of chyawanprash in India. But the one which is widely accepted states that chyawanprash was first made and used by saint Chyawan. He practiced tapascharya to gain enlightenment (moksha) for number of years, which made him old and weak. Ashvini kumars created this medical formulation for Chyawan rishi and offerd him this formulation after the use of which the chywan rishi regain his youth, strength, and aphrodisiac on him in his extreme old age, and rejuvenated his body. That medicine was named chyawanprash in honour of saint Chyawan. The first documented evidence of this formula is found in the principal Ayurvedic text Charak Samhita. According to Charak Samhita, chyawanprash is the foremost of all herbal rejuvenative tonics.

## Composition

The real recipe of chyawanprash is given in ancient Ayurvedic texts like Ashtangahridayam, Charak Samhita, Sangandhara Samhita etc. Almost all prinicipal ayurvedic textbook contain receipe of chyawanprash. Chyawanprash is a mixture of more than 40 herbal ingredients. Other chief ingredients include honey, sugar cane concentrate, ghee, ashwagandha, shatavari, bala, black pepper, cinnamon, cardamom, cloves, saffron, etc. All these ingredients make chyawanprash a rich source of phyto-nutrients and antioxidants. All the ingredients incorporated in Chyawanprash as well as product Chyawanprash are scientifically studied individually for their health benefits. The dominant ingredient 'Amla', highly rich is tannins and phenolics, is an intensely sour citrus fruit. It grows on a long living tree in Indian subcontinent. Fresh Amla berries are the key ingredient in Chyawanprash. Details of amla is given in Chapter 6. Use and benefits of honey are well known. Its antibacterial activity makes it an ideal ingredient to preserve this herbal jam for long duration. Presence of different nutrient rich ingredients in a specific quantity in Chyawanprash create a powerful synergy for optimum health enhancing benefits of the tonic which re established through research. findings. Original recipe of Chyawanprash, as stated in Charak Samhita, requires the use of fresh Amla berries and whole herbs. There are very few companies who are offering this tonic made with original recipe under their brand.

## Appearance and Taste

It is a brown-coloured, sticky paste. It has the consistency of jam and combination of sweet/sour/astringent/spicy taste. It can be eaten directly or mixed in warm milk or water. The taste is interesting a blend of sweet, sour, astringent, pungent taste, which everybody like. Most people are surprised as to how good it tastes. Chyawanprash is said to be beneficial for everyone. Accordingly, you need 1-2 teaspoon (12-28 g.) of Chyawanprash every day, preferably with 100 – 250 ml milk. It can also be used as a spread and applied on bread/toast. Dabur has lanched Fruit-flavoured Chyawanprash in orange and mango variants with an intention to make Chyawanprash universally accepted by the public and children in particular.

## Commercialization

Chyawanprash is a ancient preparation. Now a days different companies are making Chyawanprash in their own ways by removing some ingredients and adding their own. The number of herbs used in preparation of the paste varies from 25 to 80, but the main ingredient of all Chyawanprash is amla berry which form the base. Sometimes this variation in comoposition is done to market the product among children. Inspite of doing this, the product is still most popular health supplement. Chyawanprash unique taste is liked by men, women, children, the senior citizens, all consume it regularly, especially during the winter season. If the popularity of a product is measured by its sales turn over, acceptance of brand and a acceptability by wide section of societry, then chyawanprash certainly makes the mark. Its usage is also being aggressively promoted among the youth and the children to boost growth and achieve higher sales.

One thing worrisome is the *p*ercentage of sugar levels, crossing the 60% and touching the 70% mark. It appears that some of the herbal contents of are bitter, which make the product unpalatable but mostly unacceptable. Further such a high concentration of sugar will act as preservative and increase the self life limit of the product. Further there is no guideline about quantity of sugar allowed. To solve this issue, sugarfree variants are also in market.

Due to aggressive marketing both in print media and TV, chyawanprash as general tonic has got huge market and sales are increasing by 15-20%. Practically every Ayurvedic products manufacturing unit is selling chyawanprash. Even ayurvedic doctors prepare chywanprash and sold to their patients. Chyawanpash is also prepared at home as per their requirement. It is established fact that there is no way one can make chyawanprash by following original formula simply because all herbs mentioned in original formula are just now not available. Therefore strictly speaking what is sold in the name of chyawanprash is actually not real chyawanprash. Preservative like potassium sorbate sometimes added, which is objectionable. Some companies claimed to have added metals like gold and silver. Charak has not prescribed using metals in chyawanprash anywhere. They do not tell in which form gold and silver has been added. *Ayurveda* recommends the use of metal bhasmas but only for specific purposes. Due to lack of suitable quality control standards of traditional Ayurvedic preparations, it is very difficult to ensure uniformity of their composition and consequently quality standard of final product. There is a great variation in the choice of ingredients in many brands. This also explained the variations in texture, colour, constitancy, quality, ranging from a smooth paste to a somewhat grainy consistency. It sometimes affected the colour range, which varied from a relatively lighter brown to a very intense deep brown. Good news about chyawanprash is no traces of pesticides, toxic metals, steroids is yet reported.

## Health Benefits

- ❖ Many *Ayurvedic* scholars call chyawanprash as "Ageless Wonder". The recipe of chyawanprash has stood the test of time and is still beneficial to alleviate modern day health problems.
- ❖ Number of Ayurvedic scholars have highlighted the benefits of chyawanprash in their books. Their opinions vary in some points but all of them are unanimous about its power for general rejuvenation and longevity. It improves vigour and vitality. Daily intake of chyawanprash protects the body from internal and external stressors thereby improving quality of life.
- ❖ Amla berry is a rich source of vitamin C (445 mg/100g) and phyto-nutrients and so are the many other herbs and spices in chyawanprash. All of them are powerful antioxidants. Anti-aging benefits claimed due to chyawanprash can be due to the anti-oxidant effect of vitamin C. property of this tonic slows the aging process and helps maintain youthfulness.

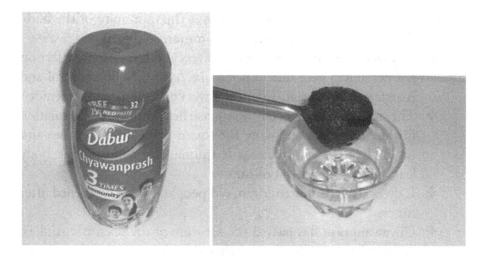

**Chyawanprash Product**     **Apperance of Chyawanprash**

- ❖ As per charak samhita, it relieves cough, dyspnea, fever, emaciation, heart diseases, arthritis, urinary complaints, diseases related to semen, coarseness of speech.
- ❖ It gives strength for children, working class peope, old age people, person weakened after illness and all those who consume it regularly.
- ❖ It increases digestive power, intelligence, memory, complexion and it helps in bowel movements, gives strength to all sense organs, and increases sexual power.
- ❖ As per good digestion and proper absorption and assimilation of food is important for overall health. Good digestion is also necessary for regeneration of damaged tissues. Chyawanprash helps to strengthens digestion, absorption and assimilation of food which is necessary for tissue regeneration and good health. Herbs like ginger, cardamom, cinnamon, amla, cloves and long pepper are used to improve digestion. It also improves the elimination of waste from the body by easing constipation.
- ❖ Chyawanprash is revered by many Ayurvedic scholars for its benefits on respiratory system. Licorice, cardamom, long pepper, bay leaf is commonly used to alleviate cough and asthmatic breathing.

❖ The rich complex formula improves the immunity of the body thereby also helping to prevent common colds and coughs.

❖ Chyawanprash helps in relieving stress and has calming effect on the nervous system due to herbs like Ashwagandha, brahmi and Asparagus. The formula also improves concentration and memory.

❖ The spices and herbs of chyawanprash help improve the circulation in the body, thus removing the toxins from various tissues and internal organs. It creates a harmonious synergy in the body leading to better metabolism.

❖ It gives strength for children, old people, person weakened after illness.

❖ Chyawanprash has passed the scrutiny of the scientific studies. A few of the studies proved that chyawanprash exhibited anti-oxidant property; hepato-protective effect in studies; reduced postprandial glycaemia and blood cholesterol levels.

❖ It increases digestive power, intelligence, memory, complexion and it helps in bowel movements.

❖ It gives strength to all sense organs, and increases sexual power.

❖ All the ingredients in chyawanprash have been studied individually by scientific and medical community for their benefits. It is not always possible to find the active phyto-constituent and the rationality of a particular herb in terms of modern scientific methods. But all that is beyond the reach of scientific proof is not irrational and non-existing, as rightly depicted by Charak, one of the earliest Ayurvedic scholars – "What is visible to human being is only a small fraction of this universe and what we cannot perceive is much more than that, which doesn't make that non-existent."

❖ The nourishing sweet taste of honey, sugar cane concentrate and ghee (clarified butter) play the important role as "carriers" that allows the herbs to penetrate deep into the tissues. It is very common to add honey and sugar in many Ayurvedic formulas to promote quick assimilation of herbs in the tissues.

❖ Chyawanprash has been in use for centuries and has survived due to the benefits that it offers. No wonder it is called the "AGELESS WONDER"

So here is to Chyawanprash - the preferred Indian elixir for many maladies!

# CHAPTER 33

## Triphala: A Natural Colon Cleaner

---

"This large and expensive stock of drugs will be unnecessary....The common resources of the lancet, a garden, a kitchen, fresh air, cool water, exercise, will be sufficient to cure all the diseases that are at present under the power of medicine." –

Dr. Benjamin Rush.

As the name suggest triphala is one of the most popular and widely used household name in India. Triphala is a sanskrit word tri means three and phala means fruits (three fruits). This formulation is originated in India, has been found to act as a complete body cleanser. Other cleansing benefits of triphala include reducing some forms of serum cholesterol and reduces high blood pressure. In Charak Samhita triphala is described as Tridoshic Rasayana a therapeutic agent with balancing and rejuvenating effects on the three humors in *Ayurveda vata, pitta and kapha*. Haritaki and *bibhitaki* have warm energy while amalaki is cool in nature. Triphala being combination of all three, therefore is balanced, making it useful as an internal cleansing, detoxifying formula.

### Composition

Recipe for this herbal supplement is described in traditional Indian texts Charak and Sushrutra Samhita. Triphala powder is a composed of a blend from the dried fruits of three tropical trees, called myrobalan plum: Amalaki (*Emblica officinalis*), Bibhitaki (*Terminalia belerica*) and Haritaki (*Terminalia chebula*). The blend is distributed into equal proportions to ensure maximum efficiency. These dried Rasayana fruits are well known as harade, baheda and amla as a part of medicine. These three herbs when properly mixed they interact and their potentiality increases many fold. Trihala as a whole is rich in vitamin C, gallic acid and tannins.

Ingredient-wise the main chemical constituents are presented in Table 33.1.

**Table 33.1 Main Chemical Constituents of Triphala**

| Ingredients | Chemical constituents |
| --- | --- |
| Amalaki | Vitamin C, carotene, nicotinic acid, riboflavin and tannins |
| Haritaki | Tannins, anthraquinones and polyphenolic compounds |
| Bibhitaki | Gallic acids, tannic acid and glycosides |

Because of its high vitamin content, triphala is often used as a food supplement like vitamins are in western countries. In fact, the benefits of this herb are so well known that a well-known Indian saying goes like this: "You do not have a mother? Don't worry, as long as you have triphala in your life!"

## Health Benefits

* ❖ Triphala not only cleanse the colon and detoxify the body, but also purifies the blood. It assists regular bowel movement. It removes accumulated toxins from the liver and other organs.
* ❖ People having low digestive fire often have sluggish digestion. As a result, *ama* is produced which is toxic substance. It is the root cause of majority diseases. Triphala ignites digestive fire and boosts the digestion process, allowing one to get maximum nutrients from dietary intake.
* ❖ Triphala contains five of the six tastes viz; sweet, sour, bitter, pungent and astringent, only missing the salty taste. Perhaps because the Western diet is so lacking in bitter and astringent, these are the two most prominent tastes for most people. As per Ayurvedic principle one must take all six tastes to maintain sound health..

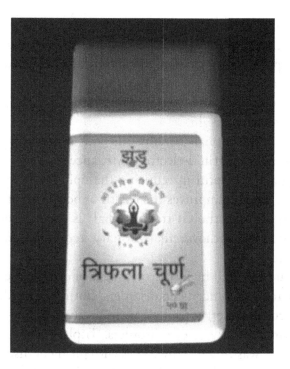

**Triphala Powder**

❖ We all know that healthy stomach leads to a healthier life. Improper digestion is the root cause of all diseases. Conversely, ill-behavior and unhealthy stomach brings severe diseases to a body. Thus, to remain fit and healthy, it is very necessary for a person to keep his stomach healthy and fit. To fulfill this necessity, various medicinal formulae advocated. However, triphala is one of the most amazing powerful remedial mixture. Triphala is excellent colon cleaner.

❖ In Ayurvedic terms, triphala is tridoshic ation, is said to have a beneficial effect on all three doshas—*vata, pitta, and kapha.*

❖ People who is experiencing trouble in bowel movement should regularly take triphala. It helps in chronic constipation.

❖ Unlike other laxatives, it is considered safe as food and is not habit forming, even when taken on daily basis.

❖ A unique feature of triphala is it provides a favourable chemical environment for the proliferation of beneficial intestinal bacteria and unfavourable environment for non-beneficial bacteria.

❖ It helps in expelling stones from the urinary tract; strong rejuvenator of the body especially for the vision, hair and voice.

❖ It helps in curing the viral infection and leukemia a type of blood cancer.

❖ It promotes one's the wisdom and intellect. It helps in reducing the excessive weight.

❖ In addition, triphala benefits the body by detoxifying it without distracting the fluid-electrolyte balance.

❖ Triphala is helpful in reducing the lipid levels in the liver and heart. Thus it improves the health of both liver and heart.

❖ In addition to the GI tract, triphala is used to support healthy respiratory, cardiovascular, urinary, reproductive, and nervous systems.

❖ Frequently used by in the treatment of eye diseases, particularly conjunctivitis and vision disorders. Both Kvatha (decoction) and Churna (powder) of triphala are indicated respectively for external and internal use in eye disorders. Triphala decoction is mainly used for washing inflamed eyes with purulent discharge or as eye drops in controlling conjunctivitis. It is a highly effective herbal combination for all eye problems including cataract, glaucoma, eye strain, itchy eyes.

❖ The Charak Samhita, one of the main texts of *Ayurveda*, describes haritaki as the remover of disease and promotes haritaki and amalaki for Rasayana, or rejuvenation of the body.

❖ Triphala has also been shown to be a powerful antioxidant, protecting cells from the damaging effects of free radicals The three fruits involved in making Triphala are also known for their individual effects.

❖ Amalaki a cooling effect that manages *pitta*, supporting the natural functions of the liver and the immune system.

❖ Bibhitaki: Particularly good for *kapha*, supporting the respiratory system as well as *kapha* accumulations in all systems.

❖ Haritaki: Though having a heating nature, it is still good for all three doshas (*vata, pitta,* and *kapha*). Is known for its "scraping" effect, which removes toxins and helps maintain healthy levels of weight.

❖ It is good to take triphala along with digestive spices Trikatu. This gives a balanced approach for cleansing both stomach and colon and makes for a good metabolic regulator.

❖ Triphala has been found to be an excellent scavenger of free radicals.

❖ Tiphala produced excellent analgesic and anti-pyretic effects without any gastric demage.

# PART IV

# MEDIUM OF TRANSPORT

# CHAPTER 34

## Ghee: World's Healthiest Food

Ghee is sweet in taste and cooling in energy, rejuvenating, good for the eyes and vision, kindles digestion, bestows luster and beauty, enhances memory and stamina, increases intellect, promotes longevity, is an aphrodisiac and protects the body from various diseases.

(Bhavaprakasha 6.18.1)

Ghee is a very renowned traditional dairy product in India and many middle east countries. Ghee, is derived from Sanskrit word 'ghrita. Due to its ability of inhariting and enhancing potency of herb, ghee is considered best among all lipid media. It is given prime importance for internal usage in diet. Ghee is mainly used in many Ayurvedic medicines and treatments. This is due to its positive effects on the digestion, absorption and delivery of Ayurvedic herbs, as well as its own healing properties. Among different types of ghees, one which is prepared from cow's milk is considered to be the best. It is sweet and strengthening in action. Buffallo milk which is quite common in India is not recommended in *Ayurveda*. It preserves eye sight, cures mental disturbances, improves memory and stabilizes intellect, pacifies tridosha. Thus cow's ghee not only is very effective anupama but also excellent food.

In ancient textbook of *Ayurveda*, Charak has given ghee the status of Rasayana. Traditionally in *Ayurveda* ghee is considered one of the most health promoting of all foodstuffs. Ghee imparts over all health, longevity and well-being. When person's digestive fire (agni) and ojas are weakened, the tridoshas are disturbed causing disease. Ghee builds the aura, builds up the internal juices of the ahar-rasa, which are destroyed by aging. It increases ojas the most refined element of digestion. Ojas confers immunity. Because ghee influences both agni and ojas is at the time it is heart of all Ayurvedic treatments. Ghee also nourishes and regenerates the body and mind, improving the overall quality of treatment. Finally, on a practical level, ghee is fully loaded with antioxidants and hence does not go rancid for a long time and remain fresh. Keeping quality of ghee is excellent.

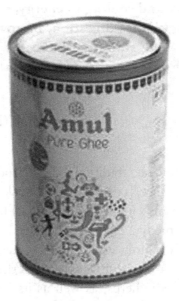

**Ghee Commercial Product**

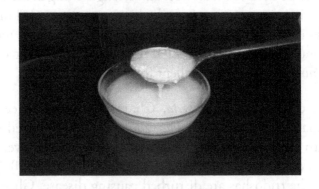

**Appearance of Ghee**

## Health Benefits

- ❖ Ghee is extensively used in Ayurvedic practice, especially in chronic, deep seated and degenerative diseases.
- ❖ Ghee ignites the digestive fire- agni without aggravating *pitta*. In fact, ghee cools the body. Ghee is hence recommended in autumn when *pitta*'s hot nature can get aggravated after summer.
- ❖ Ghee is an excellent lipid meduim to facilitate the transport of active principles of some medicine across the cell membrane, which is permeable only to lipid molecules, e.g., the blood-brain barrier where normaly transport of medicine is difficult. Ghee assists the medicine to reach certain part i.e. brain or tissue of the body. Otherwise delivary of drug in brain is difficult.
- ❖ It is prescribed for children, old and weak, those desiring good eye sight, those desirous of longevity, of strength, good complexion, voice, nourishment, progeny, tenderness, luster, immunity, memory, intelligence, power of digestion, wisdom, proper functioning of sense organs and those afflicted with injuries due to burns, by weapons, poisons and fire. Such persons should regularly consume ghee.
- ❖ It is an excellent solvent base for the extraction of herbo-mineral active principles.
- ❖ Those desirous of longevity, of strength, good complexion, voice, nourishment, progeny, tenderness, luster, immunity, memory, ntelligence, power of digestion, wisdom, proper functioning of sense organs and those afflicted with injuries due to burns, by weapons, poisons and fire.
- ❖ Ghee is one of those dietary ingredients that can be consumed by all at all times. Ghee is used in different doses for different purposes at different timings in Ayurvedic treatment. In Panchakarma procedures for the purpose of cleaning the body, it is given in larger doses in empty stomach without food. Whereas, if it is to increase the weight of the body, then it is given in small quantities mixed with food.
- ❖ If the patient is under weight, lean, bulk promoting doses of ghee are recommended. In such cases, there will be deficiency of fats and fat-soluble principles in patient. Moreover, even though LDL is considered as 'bad' cholesterol, it is required in its non-oxidized

form to build and repair the cell wall and all structural units in the body.

❖ Ghee in Gastrointestinal Tract activates and releases many enzymes and hormones in blood. it nourishes Gastrointestinal mucosa and lubricates it. It enhances the absorption of fat-soluble vitamins and strengthens the colonic flora of beneficial microorganisms.

❖ It is beneficial for the eyes and helps the functioning of the extraocular muscles, eyelids and tear.

❖ Thus, if ghee is used in suitable doses will render thousands of benefits due to nullification of toxins and toxic effects of drugs; increased absorption, transportation and bio-availability of the drugs used and also by acting as a media to dissolve and enhance the efficacy of the active principles in the drugs used. Hence, if ghee is used judiciously, ghee has enormous advantages..

❖ Ghee is widely used in number of medicinal formulations due to its unusual ability to assimilate the properties of herbs, it is mixed with, without losing its own qualities. For example, if ghee is mixed with a drying, heating herb, it doesn't sacrifice its own oily, cold nature. As most Ayurvedic formulations require heating in their preparation, ghee is favoured.

❖ Ghee not only rejuvenate the body, it is a specific tonic for the mind. It nourishes the nerve tissue and brain. Brahmi ghee is prescribed in the fifth month of pregnancy for mental development of the foetus as both Brahmi and ghee aid the development of consciousness and intellect. The newborn is also fed honey and ghee to stimulate intellect and ojas (the essence of all tissues) in an important ritul in hindu culture.

## Ghee in Panchakarma

Panchakarma was developed thousands of years ago by the old healing masters- the rishis. Panchakarma is an ancient procedure of purification of the body which is very effective at getting toxin out quickly- even those that are deep seated and stored in your fat for years. It is neither painful nor unpleasant. Panchakarma especially effective in dislodging impurities and toxins. The first phase of Panchakarma is called "internal oleation." Oleation means suturing your body with medicated ghee; increasing doses of medicated ghee are given each morning to prepare the body. The purpose of drinking ghee is to "dissolve" the *ama* or toxic wastes in the dhatus, allowing the wastes to be then carried to the intestinal tract and then expelled. Patients are also given a daily oil massage which brings toxins out of fatty tissues, followed by steam therapy to bring toxins to the surface. After several days, toxins are eliminated with different techniques such as emesis (vomiting), purgatives, enemas and nasal therapy to cleanse the body. It is traditionally considered, that the older ghee is better its healing qualities. Hundred year old ghee is highly valued in India and fetches a very high price. Such ghee was often kept in temples in large vats and families often pass on aged ghee to their next generation. Old ghee cures gray cataract, asthma, bronchitis, vertigo, epilepsy, poisonings, pain in female genital tract, diseases of eye and ears, swellings and fever. The ingestion of ghee is used in panchakarma specifically to penetrate into and then dissolve *ama* in the dhatus, allowing the wastes to be then carried to the intestinal tract and then expelled.

Ghee is used as a carrier or "yogavahi" for herbs and bhasmas because of its supreme penetrating qualities and thus ability to carry these substances deep into the dhatus or tissues.

Maharishi *Ayurveda* research has shown that panchakarma greatly reduces 14 important fat soluble toxic and carcinogenic chemicals. These would otherwise remain in the body for a long time as the body usually excretes only water soluble chemicals. Fast soluble toxin seated deeply difficult to flush out using ordinary mehods. Only Panchakarma can expel toxin out of the body.

## Other Uses

❖ Ghee is excellent for cooking. Among all cooking oils, ghee has one of the highest flash points and in comparision it is difficult to burn. In India, it is said that food is incomplete without the use of ghee. Ghee is a regular feature of Indian diet. Here we discussing desi ghee not vegetable ghee.

❖ Ghee is excellent for a gargle-gandush, to improve the health of the teeth and gums. Ghee can be used as a bath oil. Take two tablespoons of ghee and mix with several drops of an essential oil of your choice. Ghee can be used in the eyes for tiredness or fatigue.

❖ Ghee is an exquisite facial moisturizer.

## Home Remedies

❖ One or two teaspoons of ghee first thing in the morning followed immediately with hot water will promptly produce a bowel movement. It will also warm the body quickly.

❖ Two spoonful's of ghee in warm (non-homogenized) milk before bed time is soothing to the nerves and lubricates the intestines and facilitates a bowel movement in the morning.

❖ It is said that if a few drops of ghee are placed in the nostrils then nosebleed can be checked. If this is done twice in a day, then headache can be relieved

# CHAPTER 35

## Honey: A Unique God Gift

*"The fruit of bees is desired by all, and is equally sweet to kings and beggars and it is not only pleasing but profitable and healthful; it sweetens their mouths, cures their wounds, and conveys remedies to inward ulcers."*

*Saint Ambrose*

Honey has been in use for the benefit of human beings as long as 3,500-4,000 years and that too all across the globe. In *Ayurveda* honey is called "madhu". It is a Sanskrit word means "perfection of sweet". Honey is a sweet viscous fluid produced by honey bees from the nectar of flowers. One of the striking feature of honey is in its raw form is pure and doesn't require any kind of additional flavours, sweetners, colour or preservative. It is one of the best sources of energy. Honey when consumed with different natural products such as milk, fruit juices and others or can be used as jam to spread over bread. It is one of nature's most splendid gift to mankind.

Since vedic period honey has been advocated as food and medicine. It is written in ancient Charak Samhita that enjoying a spoonful of honey a day will live a long healthy life. A natural immune booster, honey is fully loaded with vitamins, essential minerals, iron, amino acids, and has many antibiotic and antiseptic properties. Bacteria can not live in presence of honey because of the presence of antibiotics and high contents of potassium in honey.

Honey is considered an "anupama" a vehicle or carrier for other herbs to increase their efficacy. It enhances their medical qualities, and helps to reach deeper tissues. Hense almost all powdered herbs are advised to be taken with honey.

## Composition of Honey

Among all foods available to day, honey is one of the most complex natural foods and contains a wide variety of nutrients. Darker honeys tend to provide higher amount of minerals than lighter varities. One hundred gram (100 g) honey contain approximately 304 calories and average 17.1 g water. Honey contains 82.4% carbohydrates, which include 38.5 g fructose, 31 g glucose, 7.3 g maltose and just over 1 g sucrose. Honey also contains more complex carbohydrates which are medium size carbohydrates containing more than three simple sugar sub units. Complex sugars are are formed when nectar is converted into honey. The average pH of honey is 3.9. The low pH, high amount of sugars and presence of antibiotics and high content of potassium do not allow micoorganisms to proliferate.

## Properties of Honey

- ❖ It is a viscous, semi-translucent liquid of golden brown colour
- ❖ Has a tendency to become opaque and crystalline.
- ❖ It has an aromatic odour and sweet taste.
- ❖ Crystallization of honey does not alter its properties, rather it sign of naturalness.
- ❖ Older honey is onsidered particularly valuable for reducing blood sugar in diabetes and for cough.
- ❖ Any medicine taken with honey is easily absorbed by the body system and recovery from illness is faster as honey has property of acting as a catalyst to the process of absorption.
- ❖ Honey which has turned crystalline can be clear and smooth again by standing the sealed jar in a sauce pan of warm water.
- ❖ If honey is one of the ingredients mentioned in a recipe, warm it slightly to fllow smoothly.
- ❖ There are many countries where this wonderful gift of nature, honey has been, and still is, used in various culinary recipes
- ❖ It is natural preservative.

## Health Benefits

- ❖ For thousand of years, honey is one of the most important medicines that has been used in Ayurvedic healing. Honey is both food and medicine, and for that reason it can be used for both internal and external applications.
- ❖ One of the greatest benefits of honey is that it acts as a transporting vehicle inside the body once it has been ingested or applied externally with herbs, making sure the benefits of the various herbs that are mixed with the honey are penetrating deep and fast into the tissues and improving the herbs' efficacy to heal and repair.
- ❖ When applied directly on the surface of the wound, it helps to remove poisons from the body by using the same vehicle technique it uses to move herbs through the tissues of the body.

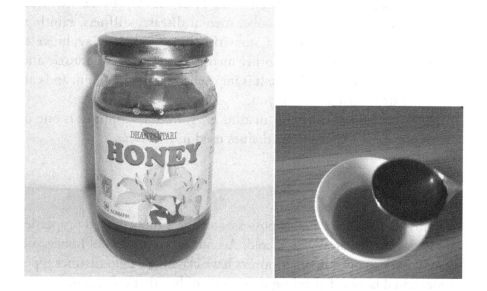

**Honey Commercial Product      Appearance of Honey**

- ❖ Used as vehicle for many drugs because of its yogavaha characters. It is also known to mitigate the increased *kapha* dosha. It should also be kept in mind that fresh honey helps to increase body mass while old honey produces constipation and decreases body mass. Cold honey should always be preferred.

❖ For individuals with *vata* and *kapha* types of constitutions the intake of honey is most beneficial, as it is warming and soothes those with cold body constitutions. It is too strong for *pitta* types, as it undergoes a chemical transformation in the intense fire of the *pitta's* metabolism, turning it into a harmful acid. Honey is not recommended for *pitta* constitution.

❖ It has been proved that honey has powerful inhibitory effect on no fewer than 60 species of different types bacteria. Many of these bacteria are notoriously resistant to antibiotics; but they are powerless against antimicrobial properties of honey.

❖ Honey can be used for the treatment of eye diseases, cough, thirst, sore throats, diabetes, obesity, asthma, and added as a sweetener that doubles as a healing ingredient in many beverages.

❖ Honey is one of the ingredient in no less than 634 ayurvedic preparations to treat incredibly range of health problems. They include tuberculosis, bronchitis, fever, kidney stone, diabetes, heart disease, asthma, colic, mental disease, stiffness, fainting, obesity, smallpox, odema, stomatitis, hicupp, alopesia, syphilis etc.

❖ Unlike antibiotics and other medications honey is nontoxic and produces no side effects. It is inexpensive, easy to obtain, and can be used virtually by anyone.

❖ Sweet honey known as madhu *in Ayurvedic* scriptures is one of the most important medicines used in *Ayurveda*.

## Types of Honey

In Ayurvedic medicine honey possesses a variety of medicinal properties and is classified as heavy, dry, cold. According to the text of honey and its Ayurvedic approach, practitioners have classified, eight distinct types of medicinal honey depending upon type of bee that collects it.

1. *Makshikam*: This honey is collected from large bluish honey bees, very light and dry natured. Used in the treatment of eye diseases, hepatitis, piles, asthma, cough and tuberculosis. Among all types, This honey is considered to be best. It is said to contain immense medical properties.

2. **Bhraamara**: This honey is collected from another type of small bees. It is sticky and transparent white in colour. Used in the treatment of urinary tract infection, blood related problems. For general consumption it is not recommended.
3. **Kshoudra**: Honey collected from medum sized brown honey bees. Considered light and cold in nature. Used in the treatment of diabetes.
4. **Pouttika**: Honey is collected from small honey beees that live in the hollows of old tree. This type of honey increase *vata* dosha and create burning sensation in the chest. Used in the treatment of diabetes and to reduce the size of tumors, and urinary infection.
5. **Dala**: Honey is dry in nature and is good for digestion. Used in treatment of diabetes and vomiting.
6. **Chatra**: Honey is collected frm brown and yellow bees that builds honeycomb in Himalayan forests. Beehive is umbrella shape(chata). It is heavy and cold in nature. Useful in gout, worms, indigestion. It is a good honey for overall nourishment.
7. **Arghya**: Honey is made by yellow bee. Good for the eyes but causes arthritis.
8. **Auddalaka**: Honey is made by small brown bee that lives in anthill. Astringent in nature. Used to treat skin disease. Also taken internally to improve voice modulation.

Cultured or purified honey, which is made by most of the authentic Ayurvedic manufacturing units as per the Ayurvedic scriptures should be use.

## Interesting Facts

1. Like poison, it spreads immediately throughout the whole body and penetrates to the deepest tissues without being first digested.
2. Honey becomes toxic when transformed by heat. It should never be used in cooking or baking as it enhances poisonous qualities that result in the production of *ama* in the body.

3. Another amazing fact about honey is that honey is the only food that will never rot. A jar of honey may remain edible for thousands of years!

## Home Remedies

❖ A teaspoon of honey and 1/4 teaspoon of cinnamon will work against a cold within a day or two! Take twice a day. Both honey and cinnamon are antiviral, antibacterial, and antifungal. Also, this treatment is a great way to reduce sugar levels, blood pressure and bladder/kidney infections, and it acts as a pain reliever for arthritis., cough, thirst, phlegm, hiccups, blood in vomit, leprosy, diabetes, obesity, worm infestation, vomiting, asthma, diarrhoea and healing Drink honey mixed with beet juice.

❖ Honey is great for building haemoglobin due to its quantities of easily absorbed iron, copper and manganese.

❖ Honey's anti-septic and soothing qualities cleanse and quickly repairs deep wounds. It accelerates new tissue growth.

❖ Honey and cinnamon made into a paste, and massaged onto joints relives pain.

❖ Try one tablespoon honey to stop hiccups.

❖ Honey in hot milk increases sperm count considerably.

❖ Honey, ground almonds, and whole milk mixed into a paste, makes an excellent cleanser and moisturizer.

❖ Daily in morning ½ hour before breakfast on an empty stomach and at night before sleeping drink honey and cinnamon powder boiled in one cup water. If taken regularly it reduces over weight. Also drinking this mixure regularly does not allow the fat to accumulate in the body even though the person eat a high calorie diet.

❖ Make a paste of one teaspoonful of cinnamon powder and five teaspoonful of honey and appy on the aching tooth. This may be applied three times a day till the tooth stops aching.

❖ An equal mixture made up of ginger juice, black pepper powder and honey when taken at least three times a day can really help prevent asthma attacks and cure asthma.

# GLOSSARY

**Adaptogen:** An Adaptogenic substance is one that demonstrates a nonspecific enhancement of the body's ability to resist a stressor

*Aloe Vera*: *Aloe vera* is one of the most widely known herbs and can be used internally or externally. Externally *aloe* helps in any type of skin problem such as burns, sunburns, cuts, rashes and scrapes. Internally *aloe* can be taken for stomach irritation as a laxative and to promote healing.

**Amalaki:** Indian gooseberry. It is carminative, diuretic, aphrodisiac, laxative, astringent and refrigerant. It is the richest known source of vitamin 'c'; one of the ingredient of triphala churna and chywanprash.

**Anabolic:** It is the set of metabolic pathways that construct molecules from smaller units. These reactions require energy.

**Analgesic:** Indian Analgesic herbs are used to relieve pain without loss of consciousness. Some of the herbs commonly used as analgesics include lobelia, mullein etc.

**Anesthetic:** An anesthetic is a drug that causes reversible loss of sensation. These drugs are generally administered to facilitate surgery.

**Antacid:** An antacid is used to neutralize acids in the stomach and intestinal tract. Herbs used for this include dandelion, fennel, ginger etc.

**Anthelmintic:** Herbs with anthelmintic agents either expel or destroy worms in the body. Other similar terms to describe such agents include vermifuge. Herbs with these fighting abilities include gentian, goldenseal, pumpkin seed and senna.

**Anti-asthmatic**: Anti-asthmatic are used to help relieve the symptoms associated with asthma. Some of the anti-asthmatic herbs are elecampane, gotu kola, lobelia, ash and wild cherry.

**Antibacterial:** Antibacterial herbs are those that fight and destroy bacteria and include alfalfa, basil, cinnamon, clove, eucalyptus, peppermint, turmeric etc.

**Anticoagulant:** Anticoagulant herbs help the body prevent clotting of the blood. Herbs with this constituent include garlic, turmeric etc.

**Antiemetic:** Antiemetic prevents vomiting, and herbs with this ability include clove, raspberry etc.

**Antifungal:** Antifungal agents act against and destroy various fungi. Herbs in this category include alfalfa, cinnamon, cloves, garlic, turmeric etc.

**Antigalactagogue:** Herbs with this property work opposite to herbs with galactagogue properties. Sage and black walnut are examples of herbs in this category.,

**Anti-inflammatory:** Herbs with this ability reduce inflammation in the body without acting directly on the cause of the inflammation. Herbs in this category include chicory, eucalyptus, fennel, ginger, licorice, marshmallow, papaya, rosemary, safflower, turmeric etc.

**Antilitic:** Plants that have the abiity to remove or prevent formation of stones or gravel in urinary system.

**Antimicrobial:** Antimicrobials helps the body destroy microbes by affecting their growth and multiplication, herbs with this ability include fennel, myrrh, etc.

**Antineoplastic:** Herbs with this quality destroy, inhibit and prevent tumors. Herbs in this category include *aloe* vera, black walnut, flaxseed, garlic, saffron, turmeric etc.

**Antioxidant:** Antioxidant herbs counteract the negative effects of oxidation on body tissues. Included in this category are barley, bilberry, gingo biloba, rosemary, sage and turmeric.

**Anti-pyretic:** This constituent counteracts the effects of periodic diseases (intermittent) like malaria. Herbs in this category include eucalyptus, goldenseal Antipyretics from the anti, *against*, nd pyreticus, *pertaining to fever*, are substances that reduce fever.

**Anti-rheumatic:** A herb which relieves or prevents rheumatism.

**Anti-spasmodic:** Antispasmodics are a group (class) of medicines that can help to control some symptoms that arise from the gut (intestines) - in particular, gut spasm.

**Antitussive:** Herbs with antitussive agents are cough suppressants. Herbs in this category include mullein and wild cherry bark.

**Aphrodisiac:** An aphrodisiac is a substance that increases sexual desire.

**Arthritis:** An inflammatory condition of the joints.

**Ashoka:** It is also used in fever, colic, ulcers and pimples. The seeds are strengthening and the ash of plant is good for external application rheumatic arthritis

**Ashwagandha:** It is tonic, astringent, deobstruent, nervine, and sedative. It is popularly known as Indian ginseng. It gives vitality and vigour and helps in building greater endurance

**Asthma:** A respiratory disorder in which there is breathlessness and wheezing sound.

**Astringent:** An astringent acts to contract and tighten. This constricting action can help eliminate secretions and hemorrhaging. Some herbs with astringent actions are amaranth, blackberry root, capsicum, elecampane, fenugreek, mullein, oak bark.

***Ayurveda*:** Constituted of two words, Ayur meaning life and Veda meaning knowledge, *Ayurveda* means the knowledge of life. Another accurate translation of *Ayurveda* is 'the knowledge of longevity.

**Bala:** It is used to reduce the body weight. It lowers the blood pressure and improves cardiac irregularity. It is useful in fevers, fits, ophthalmia, rheumatism, leucorrhoea, gonorrhea, colic, nervous disorders and general debility.

**Basil:** It also lowers blood sugar levels and its powder is used for mouth ulcers. It is widely worshiped in India.

**Bhallataka:** It is one of the most powerful and fast acting Ayurvedic hrebs. It is used extensively in piles, skin diseases, etc. Its botanical name is *Semecarpus anacardium.*

**Bibhitaki:** The fruit is one among the triphala of *Ayurveda.* It is useful in asthma, bronchitis, inflammations, sore throat, and treating the diseases of eyes, nose, heart and bladder.

**Brahma Rasayana:** This herbal recipe has been prescribed by Lord Brahma. It rejuvenates the body and fights against tiredness, fatigue, early grey hairs, wrinkling. It is the best anti-aging formula.

**Brahma:** It is the name of the first god in the Hindu God trinity. Considered as the creator of all mankind, all that lives and constitutes the mortal universe he has the universe as his body that manifests the energy of creation.

**Brahmi:** Brahmi is perhaps the most important nervine herb used in Ayurvedic medicine. It revitalizes the brain cells, removing toxins and blockages within the nervous system, while at the same time have a nurturing effect upon the mind. It improves memory and aids in concentration.

**Bronchial:** An herb or substance that relaxes constricting spasms and opens the bronchi or upper part of the lungs, thus improving respiration bronchitis.

**Calyx:** Flower parts are usually arrayed in whorls (or cycles) but may also be disposed spirally, especially if the axis is elongate. There are commonly four distinct whorls of flower parts: (1) an outer calyx consisting of sepals; within it lies (2) the corolla, consisting of petals; (3) the androecium, or group of stamens; and in the centre is (4) the gynoecium, consisting of the pistils.

**Cancer:** A disease wherein there is abnormal multiplication of cells.

**Cardiovascular:** The circulatory system comprising the heart and blood vessels which carries nutrients and oxygen to the tissues of the body and removes carbon dioxide and other wastes from them.

**Carminative:** Herbs and species taken to release gas and griping.

**Charak Samhita:** One of the oldest textbook on *Ayurveda* written on palm leaf.

**Charak:** Charak- an ancient rishi scientist, who is believed to have spent many years between the wild animals in dense jungles, which enabled him to coin his experiences in the book considered as the bible of *Ayurveda* and called the Charka Samhita.

**Chemotherapy:** Treatment with drugs that kill carcer cells or make them less active.

**Chikitsa:** Treatment, a therapy to retain balance, practice or science of medicine.

**Cholagogue:** A substance that promotes the flow of bile from the gall bladder into the duodenum.

**Cholesterol:** A fatty acid in crystalline form found in all animals oils, egg yolks, bile, liver, kidney etc.

**Colic:** Acute abdominal griping pain caused by various abnormal condtions of bowel.

**Colitis:** A chronic disease characterized by the inflammation of colon.

**Cosmic energy:** The all-pervading energy in the universe.

**Cure:** According to the literal meaning the word cure refers to the any diseased person's state of being remedied from his ailment supports or nourishes the seven body tissues. These seven tissues of our body include the rasa, rakta, mamsa, meda, asti, majja and shuktra.

**Decongestant:** An agent that relieves congestion in the upper respiratory tract. Herbs with decongestant properties include, lobelia, valerian etc.

**Demulcent:** A soothing, usually mucilaginous or oily substance, such as glycerin or lanolin, used especially to relieve pain in inflamed or irritated mucous membranes

**Diabetes:** A clinical condition characterized by the excessive secretion of urine and increased blood sugar level.

**Diaphoretic:** Diaphoretic herbs help the body produce perspiration to help the skin eliminate toxins. Herbs with diaphoretic properties include capsicum, garlic etc.

**Digestive:** Digestives promote or aid in the digestion process. Such herbs include capsicum, garlic, mustard, safflower and sage.

**Disease:** It is a condition in which one or more body parts impair the performance of the vital functions and thus bring the absence of ease.

**Diuretic:** A diuretic is used to increase the flow of urine to relieve water retention. Some herbs used for this purpose are alfalfa, dandelion, fennel, and hawthorn.

**Dysmenorrhea:** It is a medical condition of pain during menstruation that interferes with daily activities.

**Dyspepsia:** It is a condition of impaired digestion characterized by chronic or recurrent pain in the upper abdomen, upper abdominal fullness and feeling full earlier than expected when eating. It can be accompanied by bloating, belching, nausea, or heartburn.

**Emmenagogues**: Emmenagogues are substances which have the ability to provoke menstruation. They can work in a variety of ways, but the end result is menstruation. Its action can be mild or strong depending on the herb.

**Epilepsy:** Epilepsy is a physical condition that occurs when there is a sudden, brief change in how the brain works. When brain cells are not working properly, a person's consciousness, movement, or actions may be altered for a short time.

**Etiology:** It is the study of the causes of all diseases. In *Ayurveda* the cause of most of the diseases is due to the overuse, misuse or no use of the five senses.

**Febrifuge:** A substance which reduces the fever.

**Flatulence:** is defined in the medical literature as "flatus expelled through the anus" or the "quality or state of being flatulent", which is defined in turn as "marked by or affected with gases generated in the intestine or stomach; likely to cause digestive flatulence

**Free radical scavenger:** An antioxidant is a molecule that inhibits the oxidation of other molecules. Oxidation is a chemical reaction that transfers electrons or hydrogen from a substance to anoxidizing agent. Oxidation reactions can produce free radicals. In turn, these radicals can start chain reactions. When the chain reaction occurs in a cell, it can cause damage or death to the cell. Antioxidants terminate these chain reactions by removing free radical intermediates, and inhibit other oxidation reactions.

**Galactagogue:** A substance that increase milk supply is called galactagogue.

**Garlic:** Garlic is known as a miracle herb. It lowers blood pressure and cholesterol levels, provides nourishment for the circulatory, immune and urinary systems. It aids in circulation and detoxifies the body.

**Germicide:** Germicides are known for their ability to destroy germs and other microorganisms. Herbs in this category include cloves, eucalyptus.

**Ghrita:** Ghrita is a Sanskrit word meaning ghee. It is the clarified butter made by heating unsalted butter. The ghee may be stored without refrigeration and can be used for most of the preparations that need oil or butter as the basic ingredient.

**Ginger:** Ginger cleanses the colon, stimulates circulation and helps the body to eliminate wastes through the skin. It also acts as a catalyst for other herbs, to increase their effect

**Gotu kola:** Gotu kola nourishes the nervous system and helps improve memory and enhance vitality. It is known for helping the body to balance blood pressure levels and assist in the healing of wounds, decreases fatigue and depression.

**Gout:** Metabolic disease marked by acute arthritis and inflammation of joints.

**Guna:** All material entities including the mind are the composites of the three gunas, namely the satva, rajas and tamas. These are the attributes whose imbalance leads to creation of diseases.

**Haridra:** In India, traditionally it is used to eliminate worm, to improve intestinal flora, for relief of arthritis and swelling, as a blood purifier, to warm and promote proper metabolism correcting both excesses and deficiencies to relieve gas, to cleanse and strengthen the liver and gall bladder, to normalize menstruation

**Haritaki:** It is one of the herbs in Ayurvedic combination of three herbs called "triphala. It is used against jaundice, colic, anemia, cough, asthma, hoarse voice, hiccup, vomiting, hemorrhoids, diarrhea, abdominal distention, gas, fevers, diseases, parasitic infection, tumors, etc

**Haemrrhoids:** Everybody actually has hemorrhoids or piles. This is the name for a part of the rectum that is like a cushioned area well-supplied with blood. For a variety of reasons this can become enlarged, and this can lead to bleeding.

**Inflammations:** A pathological process in which pain, heat, redness and swelling occur.

**Insomnia:** Insomnia is the inability to obtain an adequate amount or quality of sleep.

**Jala:** Water, fluid.

**Jatharagni:** Fire located in stomach, digestive fire, gastric juices, and digestive enzymes.

**Jaundice:** A condition characterized by yellowness of the skin and elevated level of billirubin in blood.

**Jiva:** It is the empirical self, individual soul or the living being.

*Kapha***:** It is one of the three doshas i.e. the water humor, the intracellular fluid and the extra cellular fluid that plays significant role in the nutrition and existence of body cells and tissues.

**Kuti:** Cottage or hut or room.

**Kutipravesika:** Entering or living in a cottage for the purpose of rejuvenation.

**Leprosy:** It is disease caused by *Mycobacterium lapre*

**Lithotriptic:** These are herbs which help dissolve and eliminate urinary stones from the body. They include dandelion, marshmallow etc

**Long pepper:** Used as spices in pickles, Used for cough, asthma,.

**Madhu:** The honey

**Multiple Sclerosis:** It is nervous system disease which affects brain and spinal cord.

**Musta:** Recommended for intestinal problems, diarrhoea, indigestion, dysentery, fever, vomiting.

**Nagkeshar:** Useful in the treatment of acidity of stomach, vomiting, loss of appetite, burning sensations in the chest after taking food, blood vomiting, gastritis, peptic ulcer and pain in intestines, bronchitis, cough, asthma, headache.

**Nervine:** A substance that calms and soothes the nerves and reduces tension and anxiety. Examples: Ashwagandha, bala etc.

**Neuritis:** Infection of nerves

**Ojas:** Vigor, strength and vitality that is the essence of all tissues (dhatus). It means the life sap or the essence of immune system and spiritual energy.

**Osteoarthritis:** A slowly progressive form of arthritis, found chiefly in older persons.

**Panchamahabhutas:** The five great elements, ether, air, Agni, water and pruthvi.

**Parasites:** An organism that lives on or in an another species, known as the host, from the body of which it obtains nutrients.

*Pitta*: It is one of the three doshas i.e. the bile humor, entire hormones, enzymes, coenzymes and agencies responsible for the physiochemical processes of the body.

**Prabhava**: When two substances of similar taste, energy and post-digestive effect show entirely different action, it is called prabhav.

**Prakruti:** It means one's basic constitution which remains unchanged till death.

**Prana:** Literally meaning outgoing moving air, this is first of the five-vayu and is responsible for respiratory functions and regulating inhalation.

**Pruthvi (Earth):** An element of panchamahabhutas which is heaviest among all.

**Psoriasis:** A skin disease

**Punarnava:** This miracle herb is used in indigestion, treatment of fever, in edema, wound healing, its mainly improves the metabolism of liver cell.

**Rasa:** It is derived from the digested food and is circulated te entire body by channels. The main function of the first of the seven dhatus is to provide nutrition to all cells of the body and the plasma dhatu.

**Rasayana:** Rasayana is ancient Indian therapy used for rejuvenation. Rasayana builds up dhatus(tissues), improves the quality and quantity of life and increases immunity in the body.

**Reumatoid arthritis:** It is an autoimmune disease that results in a chronic, systemic inflammatory disorder that may affect many tissues and organs, but principally attacks flexible (synovial) joints. It can be a disabling and painful condition, which can lead to substantial loss of functioning and mobility if not adequately treated.

**Saffron:** Saffron is a very expensive spice with a mild and distinct flavour and used mainly in rice, poultry and seafood dishes

**Samhita::** Collection of subject matter, text, or document that are methodologically arranged.

**Sankhapuspi:** It is a natural tonic for mental development of children. It has been used for centuries in *Ayurveda* for rejuvenating nervous functions.

**Sanskrit:** Purified, sanctified, the language used in Vedic age.

**Sarpagandha:** An herb used for lowering high blood pressure.

**Sattvic:** It refers to the qualities that are pure, realistic and have the clarity of perception, which is responsible for goodness and happiness.

**Sciatica:** The term sciatica describes the symptoms of leg pain and possibly tingling, numbness or weakness that originates in the lower back and travels through the buttock and down the large sciatic nerve in the back of the leg.

**Sedative**: drug that calms a patient, easing agitation and permitting sleep. Sedatives generally work by modulating signals within the central nervous system. If sedatives are misused or accidentally combined, as in the case of combining prescription sedatives with alcohol, they can dangerously depress important signals that are needed to maintain heart and lung function. Most sedatives also have addictive potential. For these reasons, sedatives should be used under supervision and only as necessary.

**Shatawari:** Shatavari is recommended in Ayurvedic texts as both a preventative aid and as a remedy for a wide array of health conditions including gastric ulcers and dyspepsia

**Stomatitis:** Stomatitis is inflammation of the mouth and lips. It refers to any inflammatory process affecting the mucous membranes of the mouth and lips, with or without oral ulceration.[2]

**Sushruta Samhita**: A textbook on *Ayurveda* written by Sushruta

**Sushruta:** Founder of Sushruta School of *Ayurveda*, which focuses on surgical methods and purification of blood.

**Triphala churna:** The famous formulation. It is herbal powder triphala usually used in the treatment of innumerable conditions

**Syphilis:** s a sexually transmitted infection caused by *Treponema pallidum* subspecies *pallidum*. The primary route of transmission is through sexual contact; it may also be transmitted from mother to fetus during pregnancy or at birth, resulting incongenital syphilis.

**Tonic:** Herbs that promote functions of the system of the body usually used in the treatment of innumerable conditions

**Twak:** It is popularly known as cinnamon. It is medicinally used.

**Vagabhatta:** A famous personality in the history of *Ayurveda* wrote Astanga Sangraha and Astanga Hrdya.

**Vaidya:** Ayurvedic doctor

**Vasodialator**: Causes relaxation of blood vessels

*Vata*: The dosha responsible for all movement of the body.

**Vatatapika:** A type of rasayan therapy in which patient is treated on outpatient basis.

**Vedas:** It is a Sanskrit word meaning knowledge. Vedas are the oldest source of universal knowledge, which bloomed in the Indian culture centuries ago by rishis and holy saints. The four Vedas namely, Rig-Veda, Yajur Veda, Athrva Veda and Sam Veda have answers to mostly all the questions relating to life and living

**Vermifuge:** An agent which kills and expel parasitic worms

**Vidanga:** A warming herb used for managing all skin diseases, alleviating thirst, and rejuvenation., anti-estrogenic and, used as oral contraceptive.

**Vipica:** vipica refers to the metabolism of various organs caused by biochemical changes brought about by foods and drugs. It is directly related to rasa, but while the action of rasa is immediate, local, physiological and psychological and quite perceivable, vipaka action is delayed, systemic, physiological and inferable but not-perceivable.

**Virya:** Potency or energy of substance. It is extremely active attribute of substance

**Vitiligo:** It is a condition that causes depigmentation of parts of the skin. It occurs when skin pigment cells die or are unable to function. The cause of vitiligo, aside from cases of contact with certain chemicals

# FUTURE READING

Chaturvedi, Suresh. *Fit for Life Through Ayurveda*, Sterling Publishers (P) Ltd., New Delhi, 2008.

Chaturvedi, Suresh. *All You Wanted to Know About Diet and Health Through Ayurveda.* Sterling Publishers (P) Ltd., New Delhi,2002.

Dahanukar, Arun and Urmila Thatte. *Ayurveda Revisited.* Popular Prakashan Pvt Ltd., Mumbai, 2000.

Dash, Bhagwan and Lalitesh Kashyap. *Basics of Ayurveda*, Concept Publishing Company, New Delhi, 2003.

Frawley, Dr. David and Subhash Rande. *Ayurveda- Nature's Healing.* Lotus Press, Twin Lake, Wisconsin, 2004.

Frawley, Dr. David. *Ayurvedic Healing: a Comprehensive Guide.* 2nd Revised and Enlarged Edition, Lotus Press, Twin Lakes, Wisconsin, 2000.

Frawley, Dr. David. *Ayurveda and Mind.* Motilal Banarasidass, Mumbai, 2004

Govindan, S.V. *Ayurvedic Massage.* Abhinav Publication, New Delhi, 2000.

Harbans Suri Puri. *Rasyana: Ayurvedic Herbs for Longevity, and Rejuvenation.* Taylor and Francis, 2003.

Krishan, Shubhra. *Essential Ayurveda: What It is And What It Can Do For You.* New World Library, California, 2003.

Lad, Dr. Vasant. *Ayurveda: The Science of Self Healing.* Motilal Banarasidass, Mumbai, 1994.

Lad, Dr. Vasant. *The Textbook of Ayurveda: Fundamentals Principles.* Lotus Press, Twin Lake, Wisconsin, 2002.

Lad, Dr. Vasant and David Frawley. *The Yoga of Herbs*, Lotus Press, Twin Lake, Wisconsin.

Murali Manohar. *Ayurveda for All.* Pushak Mahal, Delhi, 2005.

Peackard Candis C. *Pocket Book of Ayurvedic Healing*, The Crossing Press, CA

Pole Sebastian. *Ayurvedic medicines.* Elsevier Ltd.2006. Ranade, Dr. Subhash. *Ayurveda.* Motilal Banarasidass, Mumbai, 1996.

Rhyner, Hans. H., *Ayurveda the Gentle Health Touch,* Motilal Banarasidass, Mumbai, 1998

Shanti Gowans. *Ayurveda for Health and Well-Being*, Jaico Publishing House, Mumbai, 2007.

Sharma, Ajay Kumar, *Elements of Rasayana Therapy in Ayurveda,* Indological and Oriental Publishers, Delhi, 2005

Tiwari Maya. *Ayurveda Secrets of Healing*, Lotus Press, Twin Lake, Wisconsin,2003

Verma, Vinod. *Ayurveda*, A Way of Life, Samuel Weiser Inc.1995

Vora, Dr. Mayank S. *Ayurveda ne Oalakhiae* (Gujarati), Navneet Publication Pvt Ltd, Ahmadabad, 2010

Vora, Dr. Mayank S. *Ayurveda:* an effective Solution, Himalaya Publishing House Pvt. Ltd. Mumbai, 2011